Addiction Nursing

Addiction Nursing

PERSPECTIVES ON PROFESSIONAL AND CLINICAL PRACTICE

Edited by

G. Hussein Rassool

Department of Addictive Behaviour, St George's Hospital Medical
School (University of London), London

and

Mike Gafoor

Department of Addictive Behaviour, Warneford Hospital,
Headington, Oxford

First published in 1997 by:
Stanley Thornes (Publishers) Ltd

Reprinted in 2002 by:
Nelson Thornes Ltd
Delta Place
27 Bath Road
CHELTENHAM
GL53 7TH
United Kingdom

05 06 / 10 9 8 7 6 5

A catalogue record for this book is available from the British Library

ISBN 0 7487 3179 2   24037583

Page make-up by Columns Design Ltd

Printed in Great Britain by Antony Rowe

Dedicated to our respective mothers
Safian Bibi Rassool and Megan Gafoor

'No man can reveal to you aught but that which
already lies half sleep in the dawning of your knowledge.
The teacher … if he is indeed wise he does not bid you enter
the house of his wisdom, but rather leads you to the
threshold of your mind.'

Khalil Gibran The Prophet (1926)

Contents

Part Six PROFESSIONAL AND PERSONAL DEVELOPMENT

List of contributors

S. Byrne
Research Nurse, Centre for Addiction Studies, Department of Addictive Behaviour, St George's Hospital Medical School (University of London), London

J. Carroll
Community Psychiatric Nurse (Addiction), Possil Drug Project, Glasgow

C. Clancy
European Co-ordinator ECCAS, former Senior Clinical Nurse Specialist, Regional Drug and Alcohol Team, South (West) Thames, Centre for Addiction Studies, Department of Addictive Behaviour, St George's Hospital Medical School (University of London), London

D. Cooper
Former Senior Manager, Alcohol and Drugs, Editor-in-Chief, Journal of Substance Misuse for Nurses and Allied Professionals, Suffolk

P. Coyne
Clinical Nurse Specialist/Honorary Research Associate, Riverside Mental Health Trust, Substance Misuse Services, London

K. Dominy
Clinical Nurse Leader (Addiction), Bethlem Royal and Maudsley NHS Trusts, Wickham Park House, Kent

M. Gafoor
Senior Clinical Nurse Specialist and Co-ordinator of Drug and Alcohol Team, Department of Addictive Behaviour, Warneford Hospital, Oxford

B. Kilpatrick
Research Nurse, Centre for Addiction Studies, Department of Addictive

Behaviour, St George's Hospital Medical School (University of London), London

F. Marshall
Business Manager, Addictions Resource Agency for Commissioners, Centre for Addiction Studies, St George's Hospital Medical School (University of London), London

L. McDonald
Addiction Liaison Nurse, Brent Community Drug Team, Park Royal Centre for Mental Health, London

O. McKeown
Research Nurse, Institute of Psychiatry, Former Senior Charge Nurse, Alcohol Treatment Unit, Maudsley Hospital, London

E. McShane
Addiction Prevention Counsellor, Centre for Addiction Studies, Department of Addictive Behaviour, St George's Hospital Medical School (University of London), London

J. Miller
Senior Clinical Nurse Specialist, Addictions Resource Agency for Commissioners, Centre for Addiction Studies, St George's Hospital Medical School (University of London), London

G. Hussein Rassool
Lecturer in Addictive Behaviour and Nursing, Centre for Addiction Studies, Department of Addictive Behaviour, St George's Hospital Medical School (University of London), London

C. Salazar
Clinical Nurse Specialist, Drug and Alcohol Team, Riverside Mental Health Trust, Substance Misuse Services, London

A. Staff
Manager, West Suffolk Drug Advisory Service, Suffolk

C. Unwin
Clinic Manager, Methadone Maintenance Clinic, Maudsley Hospital, London

G. Winship
Psychoanalytical Nurse Psychotherapist, West Berkshire Psychotherapy Service, Reading

Foreword

Drug abuse continues to increase and, as the major health and social problem of this century, remains a great challenge to humanity. The nursing profession has responded to this challenge and the field has attracted high calibre nurses, both in clinical practice and in the academic sphere. It is therefore not surprising that, having contributed occasional chapters to the wealth of books and monographs that have been published over recent years on substance misuse and addictive behaviour, a few talented nurses should produce an authoritative and comprehensive text, primarily intended for nurses, but also useful to other professionals. As I have had the pleasure of working with some of the authors, who are all leaders in their field, it gives me particular pleasure to write the foreword to their outstanding book.

Addiction Nursing guides the reader through the assessment and treatment of substance use disorders, explaining the technical vocabulary and providing the necessary scientific background material. It is written in simple language but does not assume that the reader seeks an over-simplified treatment of basic concepts. Indeed, the text presents an intellectual challenge for the academically well-versed student who seeks a distillation of the contemporary concepts underlining the basic and applied principles of assessment, intervention, treatment and prevention. In this context, the inclusion of case studies is particularly helpful as they put theoretical issues into perspective.

The multifactorial nature of substance abuse and addictive behaviour necessitates a multidisciplinary approach and the book provides an up-to-date account of epidemiological, social, psychological and biological aspects of the disorder. The varieties of physical harm resulting from substance abuse are authoritatively described as well as its impact upon the person's family, home and work and on public health. Modern advances in assessment, intervention, treatment and prevention are carefully assessed and ways of achieving further improvements in therapy and rehabilitation are discussed. Throughout the book, the fundamental responsibilities of the nurse to promote health, to prevent illness, to restore health and to alleviate suffering are emphasised; and the caring attitudes of the authors, their wide experience and their up-to-date knowledge is transparently obvious.

Addiction Nursing is a practical guide for the care of individuals with substance misuse problems and is full of general and specific information. Useful, practical aspects are covered such as how to assess the individual and his/her immediate environment and how to plan therapeutic nursing interventions and, in addition, the important issues of liaison with other services and acting as an advocate for patient and the family are explored.

In summary, this is an essential book, certainly for nurses, but also for students of other disciplines in Addictive Behaviour and will be a valuable addition to any healthcare service library. The authors are to be congratulated for so admirably filling a long-standing gap and have presented their material in a lively and interesting style, with minimal duplication between chapters. They have provided us with a practical handbook which will be genuinely useful to all members of multidisciplinary teams dealing with substance misuse problems.

Hamid Ghodse
Professor and Director, Centre for Addiction Studies
St. George's Hospital Medical School
(University of London), London

Preface

This book is about addiction nursing. It focuses on the professional development and clinical practice of nurses working in the addiction field in both hospital and community settings. The book aims to provide a comprehensive text on issues relating to clinical practice and interventions, education and research, management and the development of addiction nursing as a specialty. In addition, it aims to provide a framework for addiction nurses in dealing with difficult contemporary issues and in working with special populations such as young people, the elderly, women, homeless people, offenders, gay men and lesbians, and ethnic-minorities. The present text is skills-based and research-oriented.

Clearly, the need for such a book is long overdue as there is a dearth of suitable nursing books which cover the content of this handbook. Currently, most texts on substance misuse and addictive behaviour, available in the UK and abroad, are written by non-nurses. This book, the first of its kind, is written by experienced addiction nurses and draws from areas of clinical practice, research, education and management. It is conceived that this book will provide an up-to-date scholarly text to accompany continuing education for addiction nurses; and use as a benchmark and an 'agenda setting' from which addiction nursing as a specialty can further develop.

While the book addresses issues that are of particular interest to specialist practitioners in addiction nursing, it is intended also as a valuable resource for other healthcare workers in the addiction field; and to generic and other specialist healthcare professionals who are unfamiliar with this area of work and are likely to encounter clients with drug and alcohol problems. As Mark Twain puts it, if your only tool is a hammer, all your problems tend to look like nails.

Structure of the book

The book is presented in six parts. Part one provides the themes and perspectives in addiction nursing and examines the concept and rationale of addiction nursing; and deals with it as a professional and clinical specialty. Part two presents clinical practice in action covering areas of specialist assessment, polydrug users, HIV and substance misuse; and intervention strategies including relapse prevention, psychodynamic approach and complementary therapies. Part three examines issues and interventions relating to special populations and special problems: ethnic minorities, women, elderly, gay men and lesbians, young people, offenders, and mental health and substance misuse.

Part four introduces the concept of addiction prevention in primary care, and the role of the addiction nurse as a prevention counsellor. The concept and models of health education in relation to substance misuse, and harm-minimization as a secondary preventive health strategy are examined. In addition, issues on inter-professional collaboration for the addiction nurse are presented. Part five, deals with current policy development in the healthcare sector in relation to healthcare needs assessment, quality assurance and audit, and management practice in the emerging community substance misuse team. Part six, the final section, examines the professional and personal development of addiction nurses in relation to education and training, clinical supervision and research.

ACKNOWLEDGEMENTS

I am indebted to Professor A. Hamid Ghodse for his unfailing support and encouragement in the development of my present role. I am grateful to all the contributors, staff at the academic department, clinical staff, and past and current students for helping me to crystallize my ideas on addiction nursing. Particular thanks are extended to Professor James P. Smith, Professor John Strang and Dr Adenekan Oyefeso for their inspirations and guidance in my professional development. Finally, I also want to acknowledge my debt to my partner Julie, and special thanks for her assistance and support and to Yasmin, Adam and Reshad.

G. Hussein Rassool

I would like to thank my colleagues Dr Phil Robson and David Quinlan for their helpful comments on my chapters. I am particularly grateful to my friends in ANSA (Association of Nurses in Substance Abuse) for their support over the years and for the opportunity to reflect on my clinical practice. Special thanks also to Professor Griffith Edwards and Professor Hamid Ghodse whose teachings and guidance have inspired me both personally and professionally. Finally, I am indebted to my family, Julie, Clare and Laura for their patience, encouragement and support during the many hours spent on this book.

Mike Gafoor

Our particular thanks must be reserved for Rosemary Morris and her editorial team who provided constant support and editorial assistance.

GHR and MG

PART ONE

Themes and perspectives

Themes in addiction nursing | 1

G. Hussein Rassool and Mike Gafoor

INTRODUCTION

Substance misuse and addictive behaviour are universal phenomena and are now regarded as a major public health problem. In the European Union (EU), the percentage of the population misusing psychoactive substances in the United Kingdom (UK) is second only to Italy (Clutterbuck,1995). It is estimated that 6% of the UK population, around three million people, take at least one illegal drug in any one year (*Tackling Drugs Together*, 1995). In addition, the health and social costs from the misuse of alcohol, tobacco smoking, prescribed and over the counter drugs reveal most disturbing morbidity and mortality figures.

As the next millennium beckons the desire for new and fresh insights into future directions in healthcare provision becomes a natural focus for healthcare planners, service providers and educationalists. Over the past decade and a half, the field of substance misuse has witnessed considerable changes in the way we conceptualize and respond to the range of health problems associated with drug and alcohol misuse. Within the alcohol field, there was a reconceptualization of alcohol problems away from the abstentionist and specialist framework towards a public health and generalist model. The notion of controlled drinking which was previously regarded as heresy by alcohologists gained clinical acceptability with the publication of research showing that drinking behaviour could be modified (Heather and Robertson, 1983). This followed the issuing of Government guidelines on sensible drinking (DHSS, 1981), and terms such as alcoholism and alcoholics were replaced with ones such as 'alcohol related problems' and 'the problem drinker'.

During the same period, the changing patterns of drug use and sudden increase in the number of young heroin users heralded the development of community drug teams. These were seen as a more effective service response to the problem drug taker than the medically dominant drug dependency units (DDUs). However, such changes were overshadowed by the advent of HIV/AIDS in the middle of the

1980s, and the realization that 'HIV is a greater threat to public and individual health than drug misuse' (Advisory Council on the Misuse of Drugs (ACMD), 1988). The focus changed from the problem drug taker to the problem drug user who injects drugs (Stimson, 1990) and the nature of interventions shifted from the mind to the body and relationships between bodies (Lart, 1988). The concept of harm-minimization or harm-reduction (ACMD, 1988) became formalized and currently prevails, with other approaches, as the predominant national policy framework for intervening with substance misusers.

Addiction nurses have been at the forefront of these national policy changes and many of the clinical developments and educational programmes have been nurse led. These include low threshold methadone programmes, satellite clinics for homeless substance misusers, outreach work with drug using prostitutes, and the development of multiprofessional postgraduate educational programmes in addictive behaviour. Sadly, however, when historical reference is made in order to guide future developments in policy, research, education and clinical practice, the contribution of the role of addiction nurses may not be fully recognized.

The reason for this is highlighted by the fact that there has been a dearth of published literature on the nature of the work of addiction nurses over the past three decades. For instance, there is no known publication available on the role of nurses working within the DDUs and community teams, even though there is evidence to suggest that nurses were involved in harm-minimization work such as teaching and supervising injecting techniques in the late 1970s (Sharpe, 1996: personal communication). Historical, clinical and educational research are needed for documentation purposes as well as for empirical support in both education and clinical practice. The nature and basis of potential research could be subjected to an interdisciplinary approach. However, the planning and execution of such studies should be nurse led and should be used to advance the development of addiction nursing.

In the UK, it is evident that the substance misuse component of the curriculum in pre-registration education programmes for nurses and midwives lags behind current awareness of drug and alcohol problems. Educational policy makers and curriculum planners need to address this problem and restructure the curriculum around a conceptual framework. This should incorporate a substance misuse component in all branches of nursing and midwifery and a vertical integration model has been suggested (Rassool, 1993; Rassool and Oyefeso,1993) as a way forward. In the current purchaser/provider climate, the priority given to the allocation of resources for training and quality research in this field has been limited. It is incumbent upon policy makers, professional associations, nurse managers, educationalists and service users and carers to develop a comprehensive and effective strategy for dealing with drug and alcohol problems. Additionally, they should ensure that the field of substance misuse and addictive behaviour is not removed from the political, professional and clinical agenda.

Compared with other areas of nursing specialty, for example community psychiatric nursing or palliative care nursing, the role of the specialist nurse in substance misuse and addictive behaviour has been slow to develop and gain professional credibility. In chapter two, Rassool argues that the adoption of generic labels such as drug dependency nurse and substance misuse nurse may have acted as obstacles towards the development of professional identity and maturity. Consequently, the choice of addiction nursing as the title of the book is reflected in the development of the themes and perspectives from which the promotion and advancement of the specialist nature of our work are given due recognition. The alternative is to continue as before with nonspecific titles and become passive observers as other disciplines devise new concepts and new paradigms to describe our professional achievements.

Finally, this book is about much more than just rejecting the accusation of professional parochialism. Our rites of passage for writing and editing this book are to provide a template for current clinical practices, educational developments, and ideas for research and policy for future generations of addiction nurses. It is acknowledged, in this field, that when it comes to responding to drug and alcohol problems there are no simple solutions. What is now regarded as accepted practice may soon be discarded in years to come. Professionally, we have, in the past, been marginalized in ways not dissimilar to the social marginalization experienced by our clients. As the next century approaches, it is time for addiction nurses to assume a new and less timid identity.

REFERENCES

Advisory Council on the Misuse of Drugs (1988) *Aids and Drug Misuse, Part 1*, HMSO, London.

Clutterbuck, R. (1995) *Drugs, Crime and Corruption,* Macmillan Press Ltd, Basingstoke, Hampshire.

DHSS (1981) *Drinking Sensibly*, HMSO, London.

Heather, N. and Robertson, N. (1983) *Controlled Drinking, (revised edn)*, Methuen, London.

Lart, R.A. (1988) Personal Communication to G.V. Stimson, in *Aids and Drug Misuse: The Challenge for Policy and Practice in the 1990s* (eds J. Strang and G. Stimson 1990), Routledge, London.

Rassool, G.H. (1993) Nursing and substance misuse: responding to the challenge. *Journal of Advanced Nursing*, **18**(9), 1401–7.

Rassool, G.H. and Oyefeso, N. (1993) The need for substance misuse education in health studies curriculum: a case for nursing education. *Nurse Education Today*, **13**(2), 107–10.

Stimson, G. (1990) Revisiting Policy and Practice in Aids and Drug Misuse, in *Aids and Drug Misuse: The Challenge for Policy and Practice in the 1990s* (eds J. Strang and G. Stimson), Routledge, London.

Tackling Drugs Together. A Strategy for England 1995–98 (1995), HMSO, London.

2 Addiction nursing – towards a new paradigm: the UK experience

G. Hussein Rassool

INTRODUCTION

Nursing has a well documented clinical heritage in the development of specialties and postgraduate courses in several branches of the nursing profession. As an emerging clinical specialty, addiction nursing may be viewed as the interaction with patients or clients who have alcohol or drug-related problems. The concept of addiction nursing is a relatively recent phenomenon although terms such as drug dependency nursing, alcohol nursing, chemical dependency nursing and specialist nurse in the addiction field have spanned over the last four decades. The field of addiction nursing, in the UK, is only now beginning to leave its embryonic stage, but, as the appearance of this book attests, this emerging specialty is striving towards professional maturity.

It is evident that the professional growth and development of nurses working in specialist substance misuse agencies has lagged behind their colleagues in other professions. There has been a slow response in the development of a conceptual framework and a body of knowledge that can be applied to its clinical practice. In order to provide services that are responsive to the healthcare needs of the population, nursing activities and roles must adapt to changes and treatment trends (Naegle, 1989). The role of nurses, midwives and health visitors, in relation to substance misuse, within the healthcare system is likely to change to meet the changing health needs of the population (Rassool, 1996).

The aims of the chapter are to examine the concept of and rationale for addiction nursing, and to provide a brief overview of the historical and professional development of addiction nursing. This chapter also addresses the role and professional competencies of practitioners and clinical nurse specialists in addiction nursing and the salient challenges that they face.

RATIONALE FOR ADDICTION NURSING

The rationale for the development of addiction nursing as an academic and clinical specialty can be attributed to four major factors:

- harm and costs of substance misuse;
- policy development;
- professional initiatives;
- societal attitudes.

These factors are interrelated and assumptions are also made regarding other political and socio-economic variables that may have influenced both service provision and clinical development.

Harms and costs of substance misuse

In the UK, during the last three decades there has been an increase in the 'health-damaging' consumption of recreational, prescribed and illicit psychoactive substances across the whole strata of the society, and substance misuse is now regarded as a major public health problem.

In the UK, each year the use of alcohol is associated with the premature deaths of between 8 700 and 33 000 (Godfrey and Maynard, 1992). Psychiatric admissions associated with alcohol misuse total 17 000 annually and, with increasing emphasis on outpatient management, the true figure in psychiatric patients is probably much higher (Paton, 1994; Royal College of Psychiatrists, 1986). Tobacco smoking, by far the most important cause of preventable disease, accounts for at least 100 000 premature deaths every year, and a quarter of all young male cigarette smokers will die prematurely due to tobacco (Institute for the Study of Drug Dependence, 1991).

Benzodiazepines are the most commonly prescribed psychotropic drugs in the UK. The growing awareness of the risks of benzodiazepines and the rational use in prescribing among general practitioners (GPs) resulted, in 1988, in a fall of 23 million prescriptions (Institute for the Study of Drug Dependence, 1991). Illicit drugs such as opiates remain a growing problem and more recent drugs of misuse include ecstasy (MDMA), crack (cocaine) and buprenorphine (Temgesic). There is also a growing trend in the number of young people who experiment and use amphetamines and psychedelic drugs (Parker et al., 1995).

HIV infection, which can lead to the development of AIDS, is perhaps the greatest new public health challenge this century (Department of Health, 1992) and is a greater threat to public and individual health than drug misuse (Advisory Council for the misuse of Drugs (ACMD), 1988). The widespread use and misuse of psychoactive substances, including prescribed drugs, is associated with a substantial increase in health, social and economic problems, and these harms and costs are not expected to decrease over the next few years.

Policy development

In the UK, there has been a growing societal, professional and governmental interest in the prevention, treatment and rehabilitation of substance misusers. The
ACMD's report on *Treatment and Rehabilitation* (ACMD, 1982) highlighted the
need for a comprehensive approach and multiprofessional response to substance
misuse. They called for the active involvement of a wide range of both specialist
and nonspecialist service provision. In England, the most significant health policy
document *The Health of the Nation* (Department of Health, 1992) signalled a shift
of emphasis towards the prevention of alcohol-related problems and HIV/AIDS,
and the achievement of sexual health. It is argued that psychoactive drug misuse
is given relatively little prominence in the document except in relation to lifestyle
and HIV/AIDS (Ghodse, 1993). In addition, the aim of the British Government's
strategy, as set in the White Paper *Tackling Drugs Together* (1995), is 'to take
effective action by vigorous law enforcement, accessible treatment and a new
emphasis on education and prevention'. Substance misuse education for all health
and social care professionals is therefore needed (ACMD, 1994). Other relevant
policy documents such as *Working in Partnership* (Department of Health,1994),
Aids and Drug Misuse (ACMD, 1988; 1989) have helped to instigate the development of responses to meet the needs of the substance misuser.

Professional initiatives

Since 1984, professional bodies such as the English National Board (ENB) for
Nursing, Midwifery and Health Visiting have taken a number of initiatives in the
enhancement of the provision of educational programmes to specialist and non-
specialist workers. The strides made in professional and educational development
have been slow in uptake by health policy makers and educationalists. Over the
span of a 14 year period a number of reports have highlighted the need and recommended that education and training should be a priority for healthcare professionals (ACMD, 1984; 1988; 1990). The report of the *Substance Misuse Project
Training Needs Analysis* (ENB, 1995) recommended the inclusion of substance
misuse in all pre-registration and post-registration nursing, midwifery and health
visiting curricula and provided an overview of the principles of practice and education, standards of practice and learning outcomes. A cadre of healthcare professionals within and outside the addiction field has also been the key factor in the
initiation, planning and development of courses for both generic and specialist
workers.

Societal attitudes

There is now an increased awareness and acceptance by society of the health,
social and economic problems related to the use and misuse of tobacco smoking,
alcohol and drugs. Historically, British society has had a detailed body of folk

knowledge about alcohol and elaborate sets of social rules for regulations of its consumption (Griffiths and Pearson, 1988). Currently, there is also the recognition that substance misuse is preventable and that the harms associated with substance misuse could be reduced if proper intervention and treatment are offered. Consumer interest groups and parents are providing the impetus to combat the complex challenges of substance misuse. In the current climate, the public is demanding highly skilled care and interventions.

The above factors are the *raison d'être* in the development of addiction nursing. It is important at this stage to look at an overview of historical perspectives of nurses in this specialty.

HISTORICAL PERSPECTIVES: LAYING THE FOUNDATION

There is a lack of documentation regarding the historical development of nurses working in the drug and alcohol field, and it is not within the scope of the chapter to provide a comprehensive examination of the historical perspectives. Only a brief overview is presented.

The establishment of the first National Health Service (NHS) Alcohol Treatment Unit (ATU) in Great Britain in 1955, at Warlingham Park Hospital (Glatt, 1955), laid the foundation for the provision of a specialized treatment system for alcoholics in a variety of settings. During the next 30 years, 30 ATUs were established in the country for the provision of treatment and rehabilitation. A study of ATUs (N = 28) by Ettore (1985) found that 259 nurses were employed in those units, the majority working in a full-time capacity. Currently there is no available documentation of the number of specialist nurses working in the substance misuse field.

Kilpatrick (1993) has pointed out that services for alcohol and drug misuse have developed separately and at different times. The services for drugs began in the 1970s, later than the development of services for alcohol. In the UK, the regional units for the treatment of drug dependence were first created in the 1960s as a result of the recommendations of the second Brain committee (Ministry of Health and Scottish Home and Health Department (SHHD), 1965). Most of these were inpatient units located in psychiatric hospitals, and were usually combined with outpatient clinics. It is stated that between 100 and 150 nurses were appointed to posts within this new specialty (Woollatt, 1984).

Historically, both the development of alcohol and drug treatment services has been within the domain of general psychiatric services. However, in the early 1980s the emphasis on inpatient treatment shifted to community oriented programmes resulting in a plethora of agencies in the statutory, non statutory and voluntary sectors. The shift towards community oriented approaches began with the development of community alcohol teams. Subsequently, in the late 1980s a number of community oriented services for drug users were set up in response to the widespread use of illicit and prescribed drugs especially the heroin boom among young people.

Nurses have been the major component of the workforce working as specialists in both alcohol and drug fields (Kennedy and Faugier 1989, ACMD 1990). In the mid 1950s nurses were using group work with alcoholic patients on an inpatient unit (Glatt, 1983). In the 1960s, nurses working in the drug clinics provided interventions such as first aid, general nursing care and advice in an outpatient setting to drug users with associated medical problems (Kennedy and Faugier, 1989). The involvement of nurses in relation to the practice of harm-minimization can be traced back to the late 1960s. Nurses working in the newly established drug dependency units (DDUs) supervised addicts' injecting techniques and provided them with sterile injecting equipment to prevent infections such as hepatitis B and cellulitis (Sharpe, 1996). It seems that that may have been the beginning of the nurse's role *vis-a-vis* harm-minimization in the drug field.

The original aims and working practices of the NHS DDUs and the nurse's role have changed since their inception (Woollatt, 1984). The paradigm of care has shifted from a medical model to a biopsychosocial model of nursing interventions. In addition, the scope and nature of the role of the nurse working within this specialty has expanded. According to Kennedy and Faugier (1989), the role of nurses in drug dependency clinics has altered since the late 1960s towards a more holistic approach to caring for people with drug problems. However, in the alcohol field, Naegle (1983) argued that nursing has maintained low visibility and has willingly given up the psychotherapeutic role used with alcohol dependents and their family members to other professionals.

Over the last decade, the growing demand for increased access to healthcare provision for substance misusers has resulted in some innovations in service provision such as the development of community drug teams, alcohol liaison teams, day care programmes, street agencies, outreach work, needle exchange schemes and residential rehabilitation. Most of these innovations in service development have been nurse led. Working as an autonomous practitioner, the addiction nurse has been able to explore new services and options of providing care to substance misusers, their families or significant others. During the last decade the expanded role of the addiction nurse as a result of service development has heralded the potential development of addiction nursing.

The formal educational preparation of nurses working in the specialty dates back to the 1970s. The first course on Alcohol Dependency Nursing (620) started in 1976. The course on Drug and Alcohol Dependency Nursing was set at Manchester Polytechnic in 1985 as the result of the recommendation of the ACMD (1982) report. This course was planned and designed to reflect the multifaceted nature of substance misuse and the scope in practice of specialist nurses. Faugier and Steele (1987) maintained that 'what was needed was a course which would reflect the vast differences in theories of dependence and approaches to treatment and, at the end, produce a nurse skilled enough to work in a variety of hospital units and community settings'.

For an examination of the educational preparation and professional development of the addiction nurse , the reader is referred to chapter 23.

CONCEPT OF ADDICTION NURSING

The concept of addiction nursing is used repeatedly throughout this chapter and is the theme of the book as a whole. The title alcohol nurse, drug dependency nurse, chemical substance nurse, specialist nurse in addiction and community psychiatric nurse (addiction) are occupational labels ascribed to those working with substance misusers. Lately, a new concept has emerged describing the practice of nurses in the fields of substance misuse and addictive behaviour, with a more representative label, borrowed from United States of America (USA) literature, addiction nursing. However, the import of a concept shaped by the USA experience to the UK is fraught with difficulties. Besides cultural differences and social diversity, there are differences in the nature and extent of substance misuse and clinical practices. Although addiction nursing as a clinical specialty did not receive serious attention within the realm of nursing until the mid 1980s, it is now generally accepted as a specialty. However, the concept of addiction nursing has remained largely undefined in the British context.

Addiction nursing, as a clinical specialty, is a poor nomenclature and to overcome these limitations it can be described in broad definition. Addiction nursing may be defined as a specialist branch of mental health nursing. It is concerned with the care and treatment interventions of those individuals whose health problems are directly related to the use and misuse of psychoactive substances, and to other addictive behaviours such as eating disorders and gambling. Thus, addiction nursing encompasses the activities of clinical practice, education, policy-making, research and all other pursuits through which nurse practitioners contribute to the care of the clients. In addition, the concept incorporates the use of the principles of nursing practice, and a range of psychosocial interventions strategies including complementary therapies. The term addiction nursing may be criticized on the grounds that it is too medically orientated and substance focused. However, it could be argued that other labels mentioned above are too generic and lack the distinctive professional representation of addiction nursing.

In the USA, the concept of addiction nursing has been adopted by professional organizations and statutory bodies. These have produced two major documents on addiction nursing addressing the rationale, scope, functions, roles and preparation for practice (American Nurses' Association (ANA), 1987; 1988). In the document *The Care of Clients with Addictions: Dimension of Nursing Practice* (ANA *et al.*, 1987) addiction nursing is defined as 'an area of specialty practice concerned with care related to dysfunctional patterns of human response that have one or more of these characteristics: loss of self-control capability, episodic or continuous maladaptive behaviour or abuse of some substance, and development of dependence patterns of a physical and/or psychological nature'. This definition denotes a concept of a specialist practitioner and incorporates the diagnostic role for addiction nurses.

In the past nursing diagnosis has not been part of professional practice in the UK. However, in the light of the International Classification of Nursing Project, the nursing diagnosis movement has now reached many European countries (International Nursing Review, 1994; Lutzen and Tishelman, 1996). On a conceptual level, the definition of addiction nursing in the UK entails a shift away from the application of nursing diagnosis to the understanding of addiction nursing based on the holistic principles of nursing and caring. It is the constituent of the same philosophy that substance misuse is perceived both from the perspectives of the individuals concerned and from its sociocultural context. What is of utmost importance is the fact that addiction nursing is perceived as a caring and intervention process in meeting the healthcare needs of substance misusers. Addiction nurses are nurses who specialize in the comprehensive care and treatment of the addicted client, family and significant others usually within a multiprofessional milieu. However, what the role entails is subjected to examination in this section and the subsequent chapters. Is Addiction Nursing a specialization?

Addiction nursing as a specialization

Clinical specialty in nursing was first reported by DeWitt (1900) who described specialist areas of nursing practice. Within the realm of mental health nursing, community psychiatric nursing and latterly forensic psychiatric nursing are examples of clinical specialties. According to Murphy and Hoeffer (1983) 'specialization is viewed as an indication that the profession has advanced to the stage of narrowing its focus on subsets of phenomena selected from the domain of nursing'. However, in order to have recognition and academic respectability as a clinical specialty, the basic philosophical assumptions of addiction nursing must be identified and critically examined. Thus, the development of a knowledge base and scope for clinical practice supported by empirical research findings are some of the key features in the fulfilment of specialty status.

Generally, the development of a specialty evolves from a specific body of knowledge and specialized clinical practices within nursing. According to the ANA (1980), specialization 'involves adding to the generic base of nursing practice an organized and systematized body of knowledge and competencies within a discrete area of nursing, applied through specialized practice'. Addiction nursing cannot by its inherent and implicit nature develop a coherent body of pure knowledge and theories as distinct from other disciplines. The conceptual framework of addiction nursing is inherently a multidisciplinary business. Its body of knowledge and clinical practice are derived from nursing, psychiatry, medicine, psychology, sociology, health economics, criminology and law, public health and ethics. In other words, the present state of both the conceptual framework and development of addiction nursing is derived mainly from nursing and a range of 'borrowed theories'. For this reason, it would be futile to consider examining the existing theories of addiction nursing, which cannot be fully distinguished from the theory and practice of other healthcare professionals.

Nursing is essentially an applied science. It is acknowledged that nursing specialties, like addiction nursing, can best contribute to nursing science by generating and testing its sub-theory and expanded practice. Murphy and Hoeffer (1983), have suggested that a limited-scope practice theory is desirable in addiction nursing. A limited-scope practice theory, according to Murphy and Hoeffer (1983), is composed of a set of propositions regarding the relationships between concepts representative of at least two of these phenomena (person, environment, health, and nursing action), one of which must be nursing actions. It is argued that addiction nursing as a specialty fits the major paradigm of nursing science in terms of the individual, environment, health status and nursing interventions. In effect, it goes beyond nursing activities.

However there are inherent dangers in promoting the dichotomy between the development of theory and clinical practice if the viability of addiction nursing as a clinical specialty depends on its contributions to theory development and pay little attention to supporting empirical evidence in clinical practice. As an emerging nursing specialty, it would be beneficial to adopt a cautious stance in both contextual and theory development from which to evaluate our clinical practice. Addiction nursing as a clinical specialty needs to fulfil some fundamental criteria on the road to professional and clinical maturity. Steele (1985) states that as specialty practice matures, the basic criteria should include a specialized body of knowledge, use of generic standards, and specific standards for the phenomena of concern appropriate to that specialty.

Developing the scope of specialist practice

The scope of professional practice in addiction nursing is centred on:

- understanding the nature and extent of substance misuse and addictive behaviour (alcohol, drug, eating disorders, gambling and excessive sexual appetites);
- understanding the different health, social, psychological and economic and legal problems associated with substance misuse;
- possessing nursing skills and a range of specialists skills and competencies.

Addiction nursing is not a monolithic specialty but has incorporated nursing interventions combined with a multidisciplinary perspective of assessment and intervention strategies.

The scope of addiction nursing practice goes far beyond the traditional lines of nursing specialty. It is stated that 'addiction nursing practice encompasses an area of concern extending over the entire health–illness continuum. Inherent in addiction nursing practice is the responsibility to collaborate with other professionals and use concepts from all relevant disciplines to form a foundation for care of the clients.' (ANA NNSA, 1988).

According to Kennedy and Faugier (1989) a specialist nurse is 'the person who has chosen to work with clients with drug and alcohol problems in a full-time capacity'. This definition is vague and can be broadened to include nurses who have gained this expertise through clinical/reflective experiences and/or those who have gained a postprofessional or an academic qualification in addictive behaviour or substance misuse. The specialty of addiction nursing has tradition-ally been defined according to the settings, addiction nurses work in both residential and community settings.

In the multidisciplinary field of substance misuse, there is a blurring of roles with other disciplines. The blurring of clinical boundaries within the multidisciplinary team has meant more autonomous therapeutic roles for addiction nurses. The strengths of these nurse practitioners are that they are able to deliver high quality nursing care as well as other psychosocial interventions. However, it has been difficult for those nurses to forge a single identity 'drug worker or addiction nurse'. The blurring of role with other members of the multidisciplinary team and the expanded clinical practice are seen as a positive development with regard to the care and treatment responses in meeting the physical, social, psychological and spiritual needs of the substance misuser. Addiction requires a multiprofessional response to a multifaceted problem, but addiction nurses need a specialist identity to meet the divergent health needs of substance misusers.

Roles of addiction nurses

The expansion of the addiction nurses' role over the last decades has paralled changes in healthcare reforms and healthcare provision. These changes include greater emphasis on community oriented services and preventive health education in relation to smoking, drug taking and drinking. The roles of the nurse in relation to substance misuse have been highlighted in a recent document from the World Health Organization (WHO)/ International Council of Nurses (ICN) (WHO/ICN, 1991). These roles are: provider of care; educator/resource; counsellor/therapist; advocate; promoter of health; researcher; supervisor/leader; and consultant. The role of the addiction nurse goes beyond that of a nurse practitioner. It has been identified that there is a role differentiation between registered nurse practitioners and clinical nurse specialists working within a residential or community based setting. The prescribed roles are subjected to future empirical investigations. A sum-mary of the differing roles is shown in Table 2.1; and a typology of the role of addiction nurse is examined in the next section.

Typology of role of addiction nurses

Clinician
The addiction nurse as a clinical nurse specialist provides a client-centred approach in relation to indepth specialist nursing assessment, nursing care, coun-selling and harm-minimization. The roles of the addiction nurse should not only include the provision of basic healthcare but should also incorporate specialist assessment, planning, implementation and evaluation of the care provided to clients. They have a direct role in patient care whether they are based in a resi-dential or community setting. Prevention strategies and interventions are directed at the individual client, family or significant others. Haack (1983) supports the

Table 2.1 Role differentiation in addiction nursing

Role	Registered practitioner	Clinical nurse specialist
Provider of care	Primary care, assessment planning, implementing and evaluation of care and treatment.	
Educator	Prevention, health education, harm-minimization, teaching patients and families	Education and training of other healthcare professionals, teaching junior staff.
Consultant	Liaison with other disciplines	Resource to nurses and other disciplines: clinical, educational, policy-making. Advisory role in bodies.
Research	Awareness of current research, basic data collection	Identify and initiate research activities. Apply research findings to clinical practice. Carry out research. Publications.
Management	Management of patient care	Co-ordination of clinical care and treatment. Management of staff and resources. Personnel functions. Clinical supervision.
Advocacy	Patient self-empowerment	Lobbying for change. Community self-empowerment.

addiction nurse as therapist because of nursing biopsychosocial orientation. With this typology, counselling is an integral part of the nurse's role. A large component of the work of addiction nurses is related to counselling.

Consultant
The role of the addiction nurse as a consultant is very broad and the process is either task or process oriented (Edlund *et al.*, 1987; Poteet, 1988). During a consultation, the addiction nurse 'utilizes the nursing process to guide practice. Whether the consultation is for management of a difficult client, directing a complex family situation, or solving an organizational problem, the clinical nurse specialist gathers data and plans, implements, and evaluates every consultation' (Leiker, 1989). Consultations are also provided for healthcare professionals of other disciplines who may lack specialist knowledge about substance misuse. For example, consultations may be provided for midwives or other healthcare

professionals on the care and management of pregnant drug misusers. The role also incorporates liaison and networking activities.

Educator

Education is part of the addiction nurse's role and also an integrated component of the consultation process. It is acknowledged that most consultation processes are educational in nature and practice. As an educator, the addiction nurse is involved in health education and in educating clients, colleagues and the community. This takes the form of harm-minimization and general drug and alcohol education programmes.

Researcher

This role or lack of it has been one of the contributing factors to the slow development and professional credibility of this specialty. There is a paucity of research in theory development and research-based practice. However, there are a few research nurses working in a full-time capacity within the addiction field whose primary role is that of a 'research assistant'. This can be construed as addiction nurses providing the necessary skills in the development and implementation of research activities for the benefit of other disciplines. There are external constraints such as lack of funding, low priority accorded to nursing research in the addiction field and possibly the recognition accorded to research and the lack of adequate preparation of nurses in research methodologies. An examination of research in addiction nursing is presented in chapter 25.

Advocate

The need for nurses to act as advocates has long been recognized. Advocacy in nursing is the act of informing and supporting a person so that he or she can make the best decisions possible for himself or herself (Kohnke, 1980). Clients or patients need to be informed about their health and legal rights in specific situations and they need the relevant information to make decisions based on informed choice. The responsibility and lobbying for improved quality of services and change, and empowering people in terms of healthcare are part of the advocacy role of the nurse. Although the empowerment of consumer of healthcare is acknowledged, attention should also focus on the whole quality of life as a counter balance to narrow concentration of substance misuse. Addiction nurses have a key role in shaping the health agenda in substance misuse policy in education, practice and research.

Manager or team leader

In some agencies, mainly at community level, addiction nurses have a managerial and coordinator role. For an examination of the management of a community drug team, the reader is referred to chapter 22. Addiction nurses work in collaboration with other disciplines and assume leadership in the provision of quality care and treatment for substance misusers. They also have a key role in policy development and guidelines for clinical practice. Other responsibilities within this domain are: participating in clinical supervision, quality assurance processes, peer review. The Royal College of Nursing (RCN, 1988) has indicated that leading practitioners in nursing specialties should have the management power in influencing practice.

A working party of the RCN examined the role of nursing specialties and specialist nursing roles and identified the main roles in specialist practice (RCN, 1988):

- clinical role;
- consultative role;
- teaching role;
- management role;
- application of relevant research.

These five key roles are the essence of practice and potential professional competencies of the clinical nurse specialist in addiction nursing. In a study of addiction nurses, Rassool *et al.* (1994) found that addiction nurses are involved in teaching and supervision, are more aware of their managerial role and skills, and more likely to be involved in evaluating work practices (research). Another significant finding is the liaison and consultation role of addiction nurses with other professionals when formulating tailor-made care plans. These findings suggest that addiction nurses are developing clinical, managerial, educational and evaluative roles. This is a preliminary finding and research is underway to evaluate the professional competencies of addiction nurses.

RESPONDING TO THE CHALLENGE

Addiction nursing as a specialty, in the UK, faces numerous challenges in its path towards professional recognition. The changing nature of substance misuse and the sociopolitical reality of healthcare reforms in responding to substance misusers demand a cultural shift in many of the paradigms that have traditionally guided the work of addiction nurses. More emphases are being directed towards public health, prevention at primary and secondary levels and health education. These new challenges will have a bearing on the role and function of the addiction nurse.

A second challenge for academics and clinicians is the need for an integrated model, theory development and nursing research in addiction nursing. Since 1980, only a few research studies about addiction have been published (Murphy, 1989) and, as yet, no theory development of addiction nursing or its philosophical and conceptual analyses have been undertaken. There is the belief that a theoretical framework of addiction nursing, although preliminary, would facilitate continuing empirical work in this area. To help strengthen our understanding of addiction nursing, new directions for research are required and future empirical work is needed to explore issues relevant to the experiences of practitioners further. The research content should remain within the parameters of nursing and focus upon addiction nursing practice and the evaluation of professional competencies. The main requirement is for such research to be carried out by nurses whose work would benefit addiction nursing as a specialty rather than augmenting the knowledge and clinical practice of other healthcare disciplines.

A third challenge is to overcome the marginalization of substance misuse in nurse education curricula and clinical practice, at pre- and post-professional levels. Moreover, the development of post-registration courses in substance misuse and addictive behaviour has been a slow response to partial accommodation by the nursing profession (Rassool, 1996). The ENB report (1995) is a good starting point in the application of the principles of good practice and education, and the standards for nursing, midwifery and health visiting practice in the field of substance misuse. It is encouraging to note that the ENB report has partially addressed the standards of nursing practice and education for specialist addiction nurses, and curriculum guidelines on the education and training of specialist practitioners have been issued. These principles are a starting point in contributing towards the development of a firm national foundation for addiction nursing as a specialty in education, clinical practice and research.

Critical to the development of addiction nursing is the role of professional associations or forums. At present there are two main national associations, in the UK, that are primarily for nurses in addiction nursing: The Association of Nurses in Substance Abuse (ANSA) and the RCN Substance Misuse Forum. ANSA was formed in 1983 as an interest and support group for nurses working in drug and alcohol services. In addition, it acts as an advisor to health and social care bodies and institutions and provides an informed response on drug and alcohol related issues to the government and advisory committees.

Though ANSA and the Substance Misuse Forum of the RCN have been in existence in the UK for some time, their valuable work remains vastly undocumented (Rassool, 1996). In the case of ANSA, the association has managed to produce a regular journal, hold an annual conference and initiated a number of training activities. This is only part of the solution. In the absence of standards of education and practice in addiction nursing, these organizations should take the lead. They should also be the key players, with other interested parties and stakeholders, in the development of curriculum and teaching guidelines, clinical standards and research initiatives.

Another challenge facing practitioners and academics is the application of different philosophies and models to the approaches to care, treatment and rehabilitation of substance misusers. The issues and conflicts of the differing philosophies of care and treatment are beyond the remit of this chapter. The relevant issue for addiction nurses is the need to address the use and application of nursing models. The use of nursing models (Smith, 1994) combines diverse elements and could provide a framework to guide effective clinical practice in meeting the social, psychological, physical and spiritual needs of the clients. There are only a few nursing models that have been adapted for use by addiction nurses in both inpatients and community settings (Rassool *et al.*, 1994) and these include *The Roy*

Adaptation Model (Roy, 1980), Orem's (1985) self-care model and Roper *et al.* (1983) activities of daily living. It is argued that no current nursing model is applicable to meet the diverse health needs of substance misusers. A high priority for practitioners and academics should be directed towards the adaptation and refinement of nursing models or the development of a suitable integrated model of care which catered for the complexities involved in substance misuse and addictive behaviour.

Finally, a neglected area is the health education of the nurse in relation to their personal use and misuse of tobacco, alcohol and other psychoactive substances. Other areas of concern are the professional attitudes to substance misusers and their impact on care. These important aspects should be given due prominence in both the curriculum and teaching guidelines. The provision of counselling and treatment services for professionals with drug or alcohol problems should be part of the occupational health assistance programme.

CONCLUSION

This chapter has attempted to examine the concept of addiction nursing, its nomenclature and the importance of developing the professional identity of addiction nurses. There are challenges and barriers that continue to impede the specialty of addiction nursing from striving towards clinical and academic respectability in terms of moving beyond a subculture of other healthcare professionals. Currently, substance misuse is back on the political and professional agenda and the opportunities remain for educationalists, practitioners and researchers to 'grasp the nettle' and strive to develop a theoretical framework and research-based practice in addiction nursing (Rassool, 1996). This examination of addiction nursing is seen as 'agenda-setting' with respect to future and further developments on the part of addiction nurses. For too long we have all accepted an extremely narrow perspective of addiction nursing and, above all, we have been unable to influence those who are responsible in shaping educational, health and social policies for real change to occur. This is only the beginning.

REFERENCES

Advisory Council for the Misuse of Drugs (1982) *Treatment and Rehabilitation*, HMSO, London.

Advisory Council for the Misuse of Drugs (1984) *Prevention*, HMSO, London

Advisory Council for the Misuse of Drugs (1988) *Drugs and Aids Part 1*, HMSO, London.

Advisory Council for the Misuse of Drugs (1989) *Drugs and Aids Part 2*, HMSO, London.

Advisory Council for the Misuse of Drugs (1990) *Problem Drug Use: A Review of Training*, HMSO, London.

Advisory Council for the Misuse of Drugs (1994) *Aids and drug misuse: update*, HMSO, London.

American Nurses' Association (1980) *Nursing. A social policy statement*, American Nurses Association, Kansas City, Missouri.

American Nurses' Association, Drug and Alcohol Nursing Association, and National Nurses' Society on Addictions (1987) *The Care of Clients with Addictions: Dimension of Nursing Practice*, American Nurses Association, Kansas City, Missouri.

American Nurses' Association and National Nurses' Society on Addictions (1988) *Standards of Addictions Nursing Practice*, American Nurses Association, Kansas City, Missouri.

Department of Health (1992) *The Health of the Nation: A Strategy for Health in England*, HMSO, London.

Department of Health (1994) *Working in Partnerships*, HMSO, London.

De Witt, K. (1900) Specialty in Nursing. *American Journal of Nursing*, **1**(2), 14–7.

Edlund, B.J., Hodges, L.C. and Poteet G.W. (1987) Consultation: Doing it and doing it well. *Clinical Nurse Specialist*, **1**(2) 86–90.

English National Board for Nursing, Midwifery and Health Visiting (1995) *Substance Misuse Project: Training Needs Analysis*, ENB, London.

Ettore, E.M. (1985) A study of alcoholism treatment units: some findings on units and staff. *Alcohol and Alcoholism*, **20**(4), 371–8.

Faugier, J. and Steele C. (1987) The specialist nurse in substance abuse – breaking new ground. *Senior Nurse*, **7**(4), 36–7.

Ghodse, A.H. (1993) Substance Misuse, Health Objectives and Gains (Editorial) *Substance Misuse Bulletin*, **4**, 1–2.

Glatt, M. (1955) A treatment centre for alcoholics in a public mental hospital: its establishment and its working. *British Journal of Addiction*, **52**(2), 55–89.

Glatt, M. (1983) Conversation with Max Glatt. *British Journal of Addiction*, **78**(3), 231–43.

Godfrey, C. and Maynard, A. (1992) *A Health Strategy for Alcohol*, Centre for Health Economics, University of York, York.

Griffiths, R. and Pearson, B. (1988) *Working with drug users*, Wilwood House, Hants.

Haack, M.R. (1983) *The Patient with a Chemical Addiction. The Nurse Psychotherapist in Private Practice*. Springer Publishing Company, New York, pp. 173–86.

Institute for the Study of Drug Dependence (1991) *Drug Abuse: Briefing*, ISDD, London.

International Nursing Review (1994) News: Nursing classification moves into new phase. *International Nursing Review*, **41**(6), 164–5.

Kennedy, J. and Faugier, J. (1989) *Drug and Alcohol Dependency Nursing*, Heinemann Nursing, Oxford.

Kilpatrick, B. (1993) Critique of the Community Team Model for Substance Misusers: With reference to the Development of Community Drug and Alcohol Team in West Essex. Middlesex University. Dissertation.

Kohnke, M.F. (1980) The nurse as advocate. *American Journal of Nursing*, **80**(11), 2038–40.

Leiker, T.L. (1989) The Role of the Addictions Nurse Specialist in a General Hospital Setting. *Nursing Clinics of North America*, **21**(1), 137–49.

Lutzen, K. and Tishelman, C. (1996) Nursing Diagnosis: a critical analysis of underlying assumptions. *International Journal of Nursing Studies*, **33**(2), 190–200.

Ministry of Health and the Scottish Home and Health Department (1965) *The Second Report of the Interdepartmental Committee*, HMSO, London.

Murphy, S.A. and Hoeffer, B. (1983) Role of the specialities in nursing science. *Advances in Nursing Science*, **5**(4), 31–9.

Murphy, S.A. (1989) The urgency of substance abuse education in schools of nursing. *Journal of Nursing Education*, **28**(6), 247–51.

Naegle, M.A. (1983) The nurse and the alcoholic: redefining an historically ambivalent relationship. *Journal of Psychosocial Nursing & Mental Health Services*, **21**(6), 17–24.

Naegle, M.A. (1989) Targets for change in alcohol and drug education for nursing roles. *Alcohol Health and Research World*, **13**, 53–5.

Orem, D. (1985) *Nursing: Concepts of Practice*, McGraw-Hill, New York.

Paton, A. (ed.) (1994) *A B C of Alcohol*. British Medical Journal Publishing Co., London.

Parker, H., Measham, F. and Aldridge, J. (1995) *Drugs futures – Changing patterns of drug use amongst English Youth*, Institute for the Study of Drug Dependence, London.

Poteet, G.W. (1988) Consultation. *Clinical Nurse Specialist*, **2**(3), 143.

Rassool, G.H., Oyefeso, A. and Ghodse, A.H. (1994) *Linking Theory to Practice: The Impact of a Course on Addiction on the Competence of Nurse Practitioners*. Paper presented at the First International Nursing Conference, 6–9 November, 1994, Negara Brunei, Darussalam.

Rassool, G.H. (1996) Addiction Nursing and Substance Misuse: A Slow Response to Partial Accommodation (Editorial). *Journal of Advanced Nursing*, **24**(9), 3.

Roper, N., Logan, W. and Tierney, A. (1983) *Using a model for nursing*, Churchill Livingstone, Edinburgh.

Roy, C. (1980) *The Roy Adaptation Model. In Conceptual Models for Nursing Practice*, 2nd edn (eds. J.P. Riehl and C. Roy), Appleton-Century-Crofts, New York, pp. 179–88.

Royal College of Nursing (1988) *Specialties in Nursing*, RCN, London.

Royal College of Psychiatrists (1986) *Alcohol: Our Favourite Drug*. Tavistock, London.

Sharpe, M. (1996) Personal Communication to Mike Gafoor.

Smith, J.P. (1994) *Editor. Models, Theories and Concepts*, Blackwell Science, Oxford.

Steele, J. (1985) Impact of certification on specialty practice. *Rehabilitation Nursing*, **10**(2),16.

Tackling Drugs Together: A Strategy for England 1995–1998 (1995), HMSO, London.

Woollatt, B. (1984) Changes in drug dependency. *Nursing Times*, **80**(47), 61.

WHO/ICN (1991) *Roles of the Nurse in Relation to Substance Misuse*, WHO/International Council Of Nurses, Geneva.

PART TWO

Clinical practice in action

Specialist assessment in addiction

Carmel Clancy and Patrick Coyne

INTRODUCTION

In the UK nurses are educated and trained through continuing education to provide assessment of health needs; physical, social, psychological and spiritual, a process which takes place in different settings. The purpose of all these assessments is to prevent ill health, maintain and promote health and alleviate suffering (ICN, 1986). The title of this chapter suggests however, that there is something beyond assessment. The question that arises is what is so special about a specialist assessment?

We take the view that to a lesser or greater extent nurses are competent individuals in assessment (Benner, 1984), but may lack the confidence or belief that the skills already acquired through their basic training are adequate when it comes to assessing problem drug and alcohol use. A situation compounded by the dearth of up-to-date professional guidance or instruments available in the clinical field. These can be likened to the experience of learning to drive a motor car, passing the driving test, and with time and practice going on to become a competent skilful driver. The process should result in the enhancement of knowledge and awareness to take on the new task competently and with confidence.

The aims of this chapter are to examine the basic issues of specialist assessment of drug and alcohol use within the context of the multidisciplinary team. It will also address some of the ethical and economic issues associated with good quality assessments.

SERVICE PROVISION AND ASSESSMENT

Underpinning health service provision is the issue of policy, the source of which can be local, regional, national and/or international (Coyne and Clancy, 1996). Current international health policy recommends that healthcare should increasingly be delivered within the primary care arena (WHO, 1978), and recent UK government policies are all aimed to 'add life to years and years to life' (Department of Health, 1992). Although, targets for health improvement have been identified, these include little reference to drugs and alcohol. Specific targets have been set for reducing the prevalence of cigarette smoking, the number of people drinking above the recommended weekly safe limits, and the number of injecting drug users who share injecting equipment.

In order to implement these policies and reach these targets, the availability of human and financial resources will have an impact on whether an assessment can be offered in the first instance, and subsequently whether the outcome of the assessment (i.e. the identification of patient needs) can be matched to the most appropriate service. Consequently, it is important to be aware that the nature of any assessment may be determined by:

- the purpose of the environment/organization that the assessment occurs in;
- the background of the assessor;
- the philosophy underpinning the culture of the organization (Johnson and Scholes, 1992);
- the health and social outcomes sought by the health purchasers;
- the health and social care targets of the government;
- the possible outcomes that can be expected (Department of Health, 1996)

NURSING CARE AND THE MODELS WHICH GUIDE CARE

Nurses, like other care providers, form relationships (Khan, 1991) with their patients, assess their needs and wants to go on to make hypotheses/estimates/lists of needs and strengths, with the view to negotiating goals. Throughout their training and education they are assisted in this process by learning how to transform negative feelings and attitudes into a 'therapeutic neutrality' (Chenitz and Krumenaker, 1987). However, nurses often forget to value their training and educational background, and the consequent knowledge and expertise gained. Perhaps we should not be surprised by this naïveté if nurses themselves are uncertain or dismissive of their discipline. This situation is often found within multidisciplinary teams, where the philosophies or values of different disciplines may prevail.

To guard against this happening, nurses need to be reminded that the foundation of nursing education and practice is the nursing process. Assessment, planning, implementation and evaluation, are core characteristics of the Nursing,

Midwives and Health Visitors Act (Department of Health and Social Security, 1990). This approach is integral to most models of nursing and as such can assist in guiding our work as well as that of the multidisciplinary team. The diversity of available models view the person, the environment, health and nursing in different ways (Marriner, 1986), many of which contain concepts that are transferable to the area of addiction. In the absence of a clear model for addiction nursing and guidance generally in the field, and the clear relationship between substance misuse and ill health, there is a strong indication for revisiting nursing theorists' work and seeking ways to adapt their understandings of how best to approach this area.

Assessment as a process of change

The purpose of nursing assessment is to provide services to help clients make and maintain changes in their lives (Belding *et al.*, 1995). These changes may be social (e.g. accommodation), physical (e.g. reducing withdrawal symptoms), psychological (e.g. managing cravings) or spiritual (e.g. providing hope). There is a need to appreciate that the client is constantly changing, and is within a network or system of constant change. This often has one of three intentions: to maintain the *status quo*; to move on to a new situation naturally; or to respond to unpredictable forces. The process of change is central to an understanding of the client's overall situation at the time of assessment, and their intentions for the future (Prochaska and DiClemente, 1986). Equally, it is important to recognize the dynamic environment within which the nurse is operating. There may, for example, be staff changes in a clinic, changes in prescribing policies, service development and necessary responses to policy changes both internal and external.

In order to provide the patient with the best possible outcome, the addiction nurse must be cognizant of his/her own attitudes and beliefs about change and the objectives of the healthcare service. For example, addiction nurses may well find that they prefer the models of change which lead to abstinence, while others may feel that they need to provide care in order to assist clients to change their behaviour, by reducing the risk of harm to themselves or others in the community. Many nurses see both aims as compatible, depending upon the client needs, the available resources, and the stage the individual's drug using career has reached (Coyne *et al.*, 1991).

Assessment of an individual or family may become an extremely complex and possibly damaging experience in the absence of a well developed and successful multidisciplinary team. In an ideal situation clients should receive the best assessment of their situation through a collaborative effort by nurses, doctors, social workers, family therapists, etc. The client should have the opportunity to develop a working relationship with, and benefit from, the expertise of more than one member of a team. Since care needs may change over a period of therapeutic contact, there is the opportunity to build upon health and social gains made early in the care episode. These include such things as overcoming systemic infection, work with family relationships, and perhaps vocational counselling as well. The team must recognize, however, that the issue of confidentiality is often a subject of great concern and fear for the client, particularly those involved in illicit drug use. Therefore individual members of the team should make strenuous efforts during the assessment phase to ensure that the client is aware of the professional rules of the team regarding 'shared confidentiality', and thus feel confident to divulge personal and pertinent information within the assessment process. This issue is highlighted particularly by pregnant drug users, drug using parents, a user in employment, users working in health or social care environments, and young people – especially those under 16 years of age.

When does assessment become a specialist assessment?

A generalist assessment should identify the presence or absence of a potential or actual problem. A specialist assessment should confirm its presence or absence and move beyond this to categorize the nature and severity of the problem and correctly match the patient's needs with the appropriate intervention. Frequently, clients who present with drug or alcohol problems receive a specialist assessment as a first response because they only become visible when a crisis occurs as a consequence of their substance misuse. This situation is more often the norm as the drug user has previously been ignored, avoided or not identified by other healthcare professionals. The strategic aim therefore must be to identify problematic drug and alcohol use at an early enough stage (i.e. screening), so that the grave consequences, health and social, to the individual and the community at large can be prevented or reduced.

Screening

The purpose of screening is to identify those people who have a problem with alcohol and drug use from those who do not (Bernadt, 1991). This type of assessment is well developed in nursing, not least within triage models used in accident and emergency departments (Read *et al.*, 1992), as well as the various nursing models themselves (Roy, 1984). Before a specialist assessor is called into primary and secondary general health services, a basic screening assessment needs to be carried out, and can easily be carried out by informed practitioners. Essentially, in a basic health assessment which is performed by all nurses before the initiation of care, there must be an objective assessment of intoxication as a result of drugs and/or alcohol.

Screening includes the basic observation of appearance such as gait, odours, dishevelled appearance. Routine questions should cover the number of cigarettes smoked daily, the normal pattern and extent of alcohol consumption and the use of other psychoactive drugs e.g. over the counter drugs, drug use by prescriptions, and drugs that are used which are not prescribed. It is important to note the issue of confidentiality at this point as clients who use non-prescribed psychoactive substances may wish to conceal this fact from the interviewer, fearing judgment and potential involvement of other social/legal agencies. It is also important that any medical complications relating to the use of non-prescribed psychoactive drugs are identified at the earliest possible time, to ensure that withdrawal effects, such as seizure, do not occur unexpectedly at a later stage. In addition, clients may fear that they will be ostracized or marginalized by the healthcare team as a result of disclosing their drug use. Some clients, in their panic, may over or under emphasize their use of psychoactive drugs so as to 'protect themselves' from prejudice.

In addition to the interview, screening assessment instruments exist which can assist both the generalist and specialist. These include, for example, the CAGE questionnaire (Mayfield, 1974) and the short Michigan alcoholism screening test (SMAST) (Selzer *et al.*, 1975). Different tools and instruments which can help to identify the nature and extent of drug use include the opiate addicts severity index, and the substance abuse assessment questionnaire (SAAQ) (Ghodse, 1995). It should be noted however, that the degree to which these instruments successfully identify the true positives and the true negatives is variable, and may be influenced by both the assessor and the context of the assessment (Glass, 1991).

When the existence of problematic drug/alcohol use has been identified, a screening assessment can motivate the problem drug user or dependent drug user to move from a pre-contemplative to contemplative stage and initiate action in changing their behaviours (Prochaska and DiClemente, 1986). The screening assessment may also include additional risk assessment factors e.g. injecting behaviour, and polydrug use. The extent to which these issues may be addressed will depend on the experience of the nurse assessor, and the nature of the environment in which the assessment is carried out.

Specialist assessment

Once the presence of a problem has been established , the assessment process will help in developing a relationship with the client. It is then possible to explore the nature of both the drug and alcohol use, and the associated problems: such as social, psychological, physical and spiritual (Glass, 1991). The assessor may well seek to identify with the individual, their plans for the future, in order to contextualize the drug and alcohol use as well as dealing with problems which have accrued as a consequence. The exploration with the client of their circumstances, includes an assessment not only of deficits, but of strengths, and of current motivation for change.

Essential to any assessment or screening, is the need to ensure the client's rights to autonomy, justice, beneficence, and non-maleficence. This can best be exemplified by the need to ensure that the assessor gathers from the client, at the start of the assessment, the client's own belief about why they are presenting for assessment and help at that time. Ignoring the client's reasons for presenting by performing an assessment by rote, can waste a valuable opportunity for health behaviour change, and generally compromise the validity of the information gathered.

In this information-gathering process, it is essential that the assessor has the ability to be able to respond to the client competently and accurately with up-to-date and accurate information. This should include the physical, social and psychological consequences of drug and alcohol use e.g. legal issues, childcare law, pregnancy issues, polydrug use, fits and seizure, withdrawal signs and symptoms. Knowledge of both options for care and treatment, including different value systems, therapeutic interventions, research evidence on treatment appropriateness and success is essential. Clients need a good comprehensive assessment, by the nurse and the associated multidisciplinary team, and they need to feel that there is hope, and feel safe within a team of experienced, knowledgeable and caring experts. Cutting through fears, misinformation and 'red-tape' is an essential characteristic of successful treatment alliances. Insider knowledge of different models of care, and different service, for acute recovery and rehabilitation makes the difference between blind hope, and informed choice. Ultimately, the possession of such knowledge may differentiate between a generalist and a specialist assessor.

Specialist assessments can be assisted by the employment of different approaches: behavioural; medical; nursing healthcare; social care; psychological and spiritual, i.e. Minnesota Model (Cook, 1988). There is also a need to recognize that underpinning these models of specialist assessment, are belief systems associated with the etiology of problem and dependent drug and alcohol abuses. For example:

- physical – genetic/hereditary disease;
- social – harm minimization, social control;
- psychological – personality, learning;
- spiritual – religious, philosophical (e.g. reincarnation, concepts of guilt/sin; redemption and hope).

Specialist assessment, invariably includes an exploration of the client's social system including family, friends, significant others. Collaborative information by significant others can help the client to develop an insight into the real nature and extent of their problem and its effects on others in their personal social system. This may include children, partner, parent, employers, friends, spiritual advisors, other health and social carers.

While specialist assessment may provide the client with many opportunities to improve their health status, resistance to the helping process is well documented in this area. We know that knowledge about potential or actual health problems as a consequence of behaviours, such as cigarette smoking, often has little impact on the actual practice of these behaviours. Health belief models (Becker and Mainman, 1975) suggest that a cost benefit decision is made by clients, at both the conscious and subconscious levels, about risk, the benefits of changing behaviours, and the clients ability to actually make changes and maintain them. Consequently resistance can take many forms. Often clients are scathingly described as being 'unmotivated' when in fact they are operating in the best way they know how.

Common examples of resistance displayed by problem drug and alcohol users may include:

- secretiveness to protect others, or sources/supply of drugs;
- distancing because of poor previous experience of caring professionals, real or imagined;
- confrontational communication to gain control or to sabotage current attempt at gaining help;
- exaggeration of drug and alcohol use, both over and under reporting, to test out knowledge of the assessor, and to attempt to attain some control – albeit self defeating;
- excessive anxiety and fear, as emotions which lead to lapse and relapse, or a sense of powerlessness and paralysis;
- challenging the credibility of help by non drug-users, in the belief that they are so marginal that they cannot be helped by mainstream carers.

Following the indepth assessment, the client and a nurse, will negotiate an action plan to meet the most realistic and achievable outcome. Egan (1986), in his integrative helping model, emphasized the need to ensure that action plans are realistic, achievable, and include a fall back plan for non-attainment of parts of the plan. This fits well within the addiction field, where some work on relapse management needs to be incorporated into the treatment intervention programmes, whether this is abstinence or harm minimization orientated (Marlatt and Gordon, 1985). Thus the multidisciplinary team needs to ensure that their initial interventions match closely to the client's identified needs and expectations expressed during the assessment phase.

While assessment can provide both the client and assessor with a picture of the client's internal and external world, we need to remember that their needs can often be met quickly, and that the priorities of needs can change rapidly. Consequently, a nurse should be able to assess the client continually, process cues rapidly and intuitively (Benner, 1984; Hamm, 1988), and, with advanced communication skills, have the ability to communicate with the client and the multidisciplinary team, and hopefully partner the client towards recovery. Clearly the process of assessment is on-going for the client, the nurse and the other members of the multidisciplinary team.

Throughout the assessment interview, a therapeutic change process can occur through the therapeutic alliance. The very act of being in a room with someone who displays care, in a non-oppressive manner, is facilitative (Khan, 1991). Clients are reinforced as being of value or not by the very attitude and behaviour of the interviewer. Therefore, it is of paramount importance that the interviewer is aware of individual differences such as ethnic, gender and religion, and ensure that the assessment is culturally sensitive and appropriate. Ultimately it must be remembered that the client, and the nurse are more than the sum of their individual parts, and that there is a holistic facet to the relationship.

The changes within the NHS towards a primary care led service have resulted in substance misuse services becoming more community orientated. Thus, there is the expectation that healthcare professionals will adapt and meet the emerging healthcare need (Clancy, 1996). The following case vignette sets out how a generalist (i.e screening techniques/intervention) and specialist (i.e. indepth and follow-up intervention) can ensure a successful outcome through joint work (i.e shared care).

Case Vignette

The school nurse of a primary school, notices as part of a health/development assessment that one of the children has not gained weight, as might have been expected, in the previous 12 months. She writes to the mother, inviting her to attend for a discussion about the child's diet and eating habits. The mother attends for the interview and is very concerned about her child's welfare. During the discussion the mother reveals to the nurse, that she separated from the child's father six months previously. Both she and her child have found the separation very difficult, but are managing generally. The mother discloses that she is aware that she has been feeling isolated, and has found herself drinking earlier in the day. The school nurse introduces the CAGE questionnaire to identify if problematic alcohol use is likely. She concludes after discussion with the mother that there is some concern about her drinking behaviour. The nurse informs the parent that confidential help is available and that it can be accessed easily. She suggests that the mother might like to have an interview with a specialist in drug and alcohol use. The mother agrees, but is cautious. The school nurse further suggests that she could make an appointment right away for a community nurse to visit at home. The mother agrees, and an appointment is made.

The nurse from the community drug and alcohol team visits the mother at home. She is careful to present both a professional image, as well as a caring and non-threatening one. She explains her background, role, membership of her team, confidentiality, and the possible type of help she can offer. She also makes it clear that she can provide assessment, and possibly some help for both the mother and her child if this is sought. The assessment begins with a general exploration of current and recent events. It clarifies the mother's understanding of why the interview was arranged, including both her hopes and fears. The interview continues, with a systematic exploration of the nature and extent of her alcohol use, and subsequent benzodiazepine use; as well as highlighting the problems that the mother appears to be enduring as a consequence of the recent separation from her partner. Personal details about the mother's past, and the family are gathered to gain a sense of predisposing risks, support systems, coping behaviours, strengths and resources.

Following the assessment, the nurse summarizes the interview process, and the data gathered, and presents her formulation to the client, negotiating its accuracy. A short-term plan is made, to address further assessment e.g. drinking diary, as well as nutritional needs. In addition, the nurse explains that she will discuss the assessment with her team colleagues, clarify what other help would be most appropriate. Further assessment may be needed in order to help the client over the long-term to manage any problems with alcohol, as well as managing the consequences of the change in her relationship, and the support of her child. It is explained to the mother, that a further meeting can be held with the school nurse to discuss ways in which she can help her child gain weight, and cope with the absence of his father.

The community nurse arranges to see the mother four days later, and provides her with a direct telephone number should problems or questions arise.

The case vignette illustrates the need for special assessment in certain circumstances. Some hints related to special assessment are given in Table 3.1.

Table 3.1 Hints to specialist assessment

- Get supervision
- Use basic interviewing skills
- Ensure that practice is research based
- Be aware of the power dynamics
- Do not over rely on client's ability to be accurate about personal information
- Use objective indicators
- Do not interview clients who are intoxicated and unable to make informed choices
- Ensure that the interview occurs in a safe environment, others must know where you are, and be able to help you if needed
- Do not interrogate clients, work with what they present if possible
- Remember you are a nurse, and health is your first consideration
- Never assume that you know enough
- Ensure the client knows the nature and purpose of the assessment and its likely implications and outcome
- Do not become despondent if a client lapses or relapses, these are opportunities to build on

CONCLUSION

The aim in this chapter has been to outline the current issues involved in the assessment of individuals with drug and alcohol concerns. Our belief is that the policy direction for substance misuse generally, needs actively to include the promotion of screening by all for all, as part of the government's aim to 'add years to life, and life to years'. This review has attempted to highlight how nursing with its broad knowledge-base, is easily transferable to the specialist area of substance misuse.

Nurses are the largest professional healthcare group in Britain and, as such, directly or indirectly manage a proportion of the healthcare budget. Assessment of clients, especially screening assessments by both generalist and specialists, is the point at which cost effectiveness begins. Early identification of those with potential or actual problems, can reduce the possible catastrophic harms that can be incurred by families and sometimes generations (Woititz, 1983). Equally the iden-tification of those who have no problem with drugs or alcohol allows the oppor-tunity for reinforcing prevention, and for maintaining healthy practices. Those who have a potential or actual problem, can be directed to specialist, brief inter-ventions, such as the addiction prevention in primary care project (Ghodse, 1995) which may well reduce acute problems, and possibly lead to a return to healthy behaviours.

The models of health change are of major importance when assessing clients. This factor is particularly important at a time of outcome orientated service pro-vision. Consequently we need to ensure that the changes we make to improve the health of individuals and their communities successfully needs to be recorded and made clear. The assessment process is the first phase of ensuring that comprehen-sive, comparable and valid data is collected in a systematic manner, to allow future successes to be identified, and to evaluate the appropriateness and relative success of different interventions.

REFERENCES

Becker, M.H. and Maiman, L.A. (1975) Sociobehavioural determination of compliance with health and medical care recommendations. *Medical Care*, **13**(1), 10–24.

Belding, M.A., Iguchi, M.Y., Lamb, R.G. *et al.* (1995) Stages and processes of change among polydrug users in methadone treatment. *Drug and alcohol Dependence*, **39**(1), 45–53.

Benner, P. (1984) *From novice to expert: excellence and power in clinical nursing practice*, Addison-Wesley, London.

Bernadt, M. (1991) Screening and early detection of alcohol problems, in *The International Handbook of Addiction Behaviours*, (ed. I.B. Glass), Tavistock/Routledge, London.

Chenitz, W.C. and Krumenaker, C. (1987) The nurse in a methadone maintenance clinic; revisited. *Journal of Psychosocial Nursing*, **25**(11), 13–17.

Clancy, C. (1996) Youth, Drugs and Alcohol – the best years of their lives? *British Journal of Community Health Nursing*, **1**(3), (In press).

Cook, C.C. (1988) The Minnesota Model in the Management of Drug and Alcohol Dependency: Miracle, Method or Myth? Part 1, The Philosophy and the Programme. *British Journal of Addiction*, **83**(6), 625–34.

Coyne, P., Wilson, D. and Jackesley, H. (1991) *Nursing and Aids: drug misuse*, HMSO, London. (Booklet accompanying the video).

Coyne, P. and Clancy, C. (1996) Out of sight, out of mind, in *Aids: The Nursing Response*, (eds. J. Faugier and I. Hicken), Chapman & Hall, London.

Department of Health and Social Security (1990) *The Nurses, Midwives and Health Visitors Act 1979*, HMSO, London.

Department of Health (1992) *The Health of the Nation*, HMSO, London.

Department of Health (1996) *The Task Force to Review Services for Drug Misusers. Report of an independent Review of Drug Treatment Services in England*, HMSO, London.

Egan, G. (1986) *The Skilled Helper: a systematic approach to effective helping*, 2nd edn, Brooks/Cole, California.

Ghodse, A.H. (1995) *Drugs and Addictive Behaviours: a guide to treatment*, 2nd edn, Blackwell Science, Oxford.

Glass, I.B. (1991) *The International Handbook of Addiction Behaviours*, Tavistock/Routledge, London.

Hamm, R.M. (1988) Clinical Intuition and Clinical Analysis: expertise and the cognitive continuum, in *Professional Judgment* (eds, J. Dowie and A. Elstein), Cambridge University Press, Cambridge.

International Council of Nurses (1986) *Report on the Regulation of Nursing*, ICN, Geneva.

Johnson, G. and Scholes, K. (1992) *Exploring Corporate Strategy*, 3rd edn, Prentice-Hall, London.

Khan, M. (1991) *Between Therapist and Client: The new relationship*, Freeman, New York.

Marlatt, G.A. and Gordon, J.R. (1985) *Relapse Prevention: Maintenance strategy in the treatment of addictive behaviours*, Guilford Press, New York.

Marriner, A. (1986) *Nursing Theorists and their Theories*, Mosby, St Louis.

Mayfield, D., McLeod, G. and Hall, P. (1974) The CAGE Questionnaire: validation of a new alcoholism screening instrument. *American Journal of Psychiatry*, **131**(10), 1121–3.

Prochaska, J.O. and DiClemente, C.C. (1986) Towards a comprehensive model of change, in *Treating Addictive Behaviours: Process of Change* (eds W.R. Miller and N. Heather), Plenum Press, New York.

Read, S., George, S., Westlake, L. *et al.* (1992) Piloting and evaluation of triage. *International Journal Of Nursing Studies*, **29**(3), 275–88.

Roy, C. (1984) *Introduction to Nursing: An adaptation model*, 2nd edn, Prentice-Hall, New Jersey.

Selzer, M.S., Vinokur, A. and Rooijien, E.V. (1975) A self-administered Short Michigan Alcoholism Screening Test (SMAST). *Journal of Studies on Alcohol*, **36**(1), 117–26.

Woititz, J.G. (1983) *Adult Children of Alcoholics*, Health Communications Inc., Deerfield Beach.

WHO (1978) *Primary Health Care: Report of the primary healthcare conference*, Alma-Ata, WHO, Geneva.

4 Polydrug users and nursing interventions

Mike Gafoor

INTRODUCTION

Polydrug use is a common feature of drug taking and, of those clients presenting for treatment, the polydrug user is more likely to be the norm than the exception. The term polydrug use refers to a pattern of drug taking which involves the use of more than one drug taken either concomitantly or in rapid sequence (Drug Scenes, 1987). Drugs such as cannabis, amphetamines, opiates and benzodiazepines are frequently used in various combinations either to boost the effect of a particular drug of choice or to ameliorate side effects or withdrawal symptoms if the preferred drug is either reduced or unavailable. However, multiple drug use cannot simply be explained in terms of pharmacology. The social and cultural meanings attached to different kinds of drugs may dictate how and when a particular drug is used. For example, so called dance drugs like ecstasy, LSD and amphetamines have become part of a distinctive youth culture with shared social norms for music, fashion, language and beliefs. Benzodiazepines are popular among drug users for their effects in the relief of withdrawal symptoms, sleep disturbances and anxiety. Compared to illegal drugs like heroin and cocaine, they are relatively cheap and easy to obtain.

Polydrug users as a group are generally regarded as more difficult to treat in so far as they have been shown to manifest greater levels of physical, social and psychological impairment (Darke *et al.*, 1993). In addition, because of the nature of their drug problems, they are likely to display drug-seeking behaviours; and to present in states of intoxication or withdrawal. Yet, there is surprisingly little clinical information available that specifically addresses the complex needs of the polydrug user (Ghodse, 1994). Most addiction textbooks tend to describe drug problems in a narrow and substance specific way as if somehow drug use occurs sequentially. Polydrug use is not an homogeneous phenomenon and there are regional differences, with various combinations of drugs used in different ways by different subgroups. In some parts of the country, for example, cannabis, LSD, ecstasy and amphetamine use by younger drug users might predominate as the main pattern of drug use; while in other areas the use of alcohol, benzodiazepines and opiates among older drug users will be a more common problem.

This chapter will provide an overview of the nature and extent of polydrug use, particularly the use of benzodiazepines. It will also highlight the main problems experienced by this group of clients, and describe the intervention strategies used in the treatment and management of the polydrug user.

NATURE AND EXTENT OF POLYDRUG USE

The use of benzodiazepines among drug users is widespread, and studies carried out in the UK and abroad have found that between 37% and 50% of drug users seeking help admit to regular use of drugs such as diazepam, temazepam and nitrazepam (Perera *et al.*, 1987; Du Pont, 1988; Darke *et al.*,1993). Recently there have been concerns over the injecting of benzodiazepines particularly temazepam and a link with increased HIV risk-taking behaviour (Klee *et al.*, 1990; Darke *et al.*, 1993). In Scotland and other parts of the UK, benzodiazepine use has been associated with a number of drug-related deaths and medical complications caused by injecting the contents of temazepam capsules or 'jellies' (Hammersley *et al.*, 1995; Ruben and Morrison,1992). In an effort to limit the use, misuse and availability of temazepam , the government has recently passed new legislation banning the prescribing of capsules and making the possession of temazepam without a prescription an offence which carries up to two years imprisonment.

PROBLEMS ASSOCIATED WITH POLYDRUG USE

Drug overdoses involving the combined use of central nervous system (CNS) depressant drugs and alcohol are a common problem for many polydrug users, and the accident and emergency department becomes another stop on their hazardous journey of substance misuse. For many, a drug overdose is unintentional and may follow a bout of heavy drinking and a lack of knowledge about the cumulative effects of alcohol with sedative type drugs. Other factors such as the level of purity of street heroin and duration of drug use are also implicated in accidental deaths from opiate use. In Glasgow, it has been estimated that up to 46% of injecting drug users die from accidental opiate overdose (Frischer *et al.*, 1993).

Since short-term memory is impaired by benzodiazepine abuse (Curran,1986), it is also common for many clients to have simply forgotten how much and what drug was previously taken. However it has been estimated that between 10% and 15% of CNS depressant abusers commit suicide (Schukit and Monteiro,1988) and it is likely that many drug overdoses are deliberate. Higher levels of depression have been found in polydrug users than in other clients (Darke *et al.*, 1993) and it is frequently associated with long term use of CNS depressant drugs and stimulants withdrawal. Depressive reactions may also follow benzodiazepine withdrawal (Petursson and Lader, 1984) and among opiate users, Dackis and Marks (1983) found that 17% were clinically depressed on initial presentation. Following detoxification, this was increased to 32%.

Benzodiazepine polydrug users are a high risk group for HIV infection. Klee *et al.* (1990) found that polydrug use including temazepam use was associated with increased sharing of injecting equipment and unsafe sexual practices. In her study of 303 injecting drug users, 90% were polydrug users with 25% injecting temazepam. The injecting of temazepam gel-filled capsules also causes problems with venous access, and complications such as deep vein thrombosis and abscesses are common. Convulsions may occur in some clients with a history of chronic abuse of sedatives (e.g. barbiturates, benzodiazepines) or stimulants such as cocaine and amphetamines. Where a history of fits is indicated, withdrawal from drugs should be carried out within an inpatient setting. Irritability, restlessness and anxiety may occur with intoxication or withdrawal from sedatives, stimulants or opiate drugs and this can sometimes lead to aggressive or hostile behaviour. Also, the disinhibiting effect of benzodiazepines and alcohol can make some clients become verbally or physically aggressive. Some heavy users of cannabis, cocaine and amphetamines may experience paranoid ideas or develop a psychotic episode that resembles paranoid schizophrenia and is characterized by delusions and hallucinations of a persecutory type.

Summary of problems

The problems associated with polydrug use can be summarized:

- depression and suicide;
- overdoses;
- increased risk of infections (i.e. hepatitis, HIV, thrombophlebitis, septicaemia);
- memory impairment, epileptic fits;
- violent and aggressive behaviour, psychotic episodes.

NURSING INTERVENTIONS

Assessment

It is widely acknowledged by clinicians working in the field of substance misuse that the assessment process is, therapeutically, one of the most important forms of interventions (chapter 3). For the majority of clients seeking help for the first time in their drugtaking career, they are usually ambivalent about committing themselves to treatment and the way in which the initial assessment is conducted might well determine whether they remain in treatment. A good nursing assessment is one that is client-centred and focuses on the individual's own strengths and perceptions of what is required to overcome their difficulties. It should not be a process of asking a series of preset questions aimed at identifying an underlying pathology (for example, personality disorder) or coming up with a theoretical diagnosis that is recorded in the notes for an academic debate in a clinical review meeting.

In the case of polydrug users, careful and detailed assessment is essential for them to receive the most appropriate treatments and therapeutic interventions which will address their physical, social and psychological needs. Because these clients are involved in multiple drugtaking, it is necessary to ascertain which drugs they are physically and/or psychologically dependent upon as well as the severity of dependence. This is usually determined by the duration and the type and quantity of drugs taken in the preceding months, together with the nature and severity of withdrawal symptoms. Observation of signs of withdrawal and intoxication, as well as urinalysis results and collateral information obtained, with the client's consent, from relatives would aid the assessment process. In the context of HIV infection, it is important to establish the extent of current or past risk-taking behaviour regarding sexual and injecting practices. Finally, the assessment process, should provide an opportunity to educate the client on the complications of multiple drug use and to advise them on the range of treatments and therapeutic interventions that are available.

The use of motivational interviewing techniques could help to shift a client's ambivalence and encourage future attendance. This form of intervention, which invites clients to explore both the positive and negative aspects of their drug use, has recently been shown to be effective in engaging drug users in treatment (Saunders *et al.*, 1995). This is crucially important since, without it, the treatment on offer becomes meaningless, no matter how sophisticated it might be.

Health advice – HIV and hepatitis

As a result of their chaotic lifestyles, increased needle sharing and unsafe sexual practices, polydrug users who inject are more susceptible to HIV infection and hepatitis B and C. Therefore, it is vital that information on HIV infection and transmission is provided at the earliest opportunity since the number of polydrug users who drop out of treatment is alarmingly high. In addition, clients should be provided with sterile injecting equipment and condoms or, at the very least, told where such items are readily available. Advice regarding the adverse effects of various drugs especially when taken together or with alcohol should be given in view of the risk of accidental overdose.

Psychosocial support

Psychological help in the form of counselling, anxiety and stress management and social skills training may be used in dealing with problems that may underlie or result from polydrug use. Counselling can help clients to stabilize their drug use or to become drug free by providing an opportunity to resolve emotional conflicts and enhancing self-esteem. Social support should also be provided to deal with any practical issues such as employment, housing and child care. Many polydrug users will experience legal difficulties, and liaising with probation officers and solicitors will help to allay their anxieties and to make positive lifestyle changes. Anxiety management and social skills training provided either individually or in groups may help some clients to deal with specific circumstances and situations that make them vulnerable to drug use. In cases, where there is evidence of a persistent mood disorder or abnormal beliefs, a psychiatric assessment should be undertaken to identify any psychiatric disorders.

Clients who wish to become drug free but lack the personal and social resources to achieve this in a community setting, should be considered for referral to an appropriate residential rehabilitation. However careful planning is required to ensure that the client is admitted immediately into rehabilitation facility following detoxification.

CLINICAL MANAGEMENT

Prescribing

The prescribing of medication plays an important part in the treatment and management of polydrug users, although its importance is often over exaggerated by a group of clients commonly involved in drug seeking behaviour. A prescription that is provided in haste and at the client's request may compound his or her drug problem by introducing yet another drug to be abused. Conversely, an over cautious or inflexible prescribing policy could lead to clients feeling dissatisfied with the service and dropping out of the treatment process. Polydrug users as a rule are not used to taking medication as prescribed and before issuing a prescription, the addiction nurse should see that the necessary safeguards are in place so as to minimize the risks of abuse and to ensure that maximum benefit is gained. For example, the nurse could arrange for the daily collection of medication from a pharmacist, health centre, day hospital or outpatient department. The assistance of a partner, relatives or friends could also be used in supervised administration of medication.

The well-known maxim of 'first do no harm' should be the guiding principle in the issuing of a prescription and this should always be part of a well designed care plan with clearly defined goals such as the achievement of health and social gains.

Types of medication

The amount and types of medication prescribed will depend largely on the outcome of a detailed assessment that should include urinalysis results. This should reveal the degree of physical dependence along with the nature and severity of withdrawal symptoms. CNS depressant drugs such as benzodiazepines, chlormethiazole, barbiturates and alcohol have similar pharmacological effects on the brain and manifest a similar withdrawal syndrome characterized by tremors, nausea, vomiting, rebound anxiety and in some instances perceptual disturbances and fits. The use of a long-acting benzodiazepine drug such as diazepam (valium) or chlordiazepoxide (librium) is widely recommended by clinicians in the relief of withdrawal symptoms associated with CNS depressants as they are less toxic to the liver, easier to titrate and reduce the risk of fits.

The prescribing of dexamphetamine tablets is sometimes indicated as a means of attracting amphetamine and cocaine users into treatment and to encourage a change from injecting to oral drug use. However, the ACMD (1993) advised caution in prescribing stimulant drugs and suggests only short-term use. Careful monitoring of injection sites should be carried out to ensure that tablets are not crushed and injected, and that the prescription is achieving its aim.

Desipramine, a tricylic antidepressant drug has been found to be effective in reducing craving among regular cocaine users by its actions on dopamine receptors (Gawin et al., 1989). A starting dose of 50mgm daily and increasing to 200mgm daily by the fourth day has been recommended.

Methadone is the most commonly used drug, either for detoxification or maintenance purposes, in opiate addiction. It is good clinical practice to establish whether there is physical dependency to opiates before prescribing methadone to a client. However, the assessment process for this could take several days and usually involves regular visits to the drug clinic for urine testing and observation of opiate withdrawal. It is known from clinical experience that many polydrug users drop out of treatment during the assessment phase, and a quicker method of assessing for opiate dependence is to give a Naloxone challenge. This is a medical procedure and should be carried out in hospital. It involves giving the drug Naloxone (an opiate antagonist) by injection and observing for objective signs of opiate withdrawal. Methadone is given in regular doses of 10–20mgm over a 24-hour period until the client is stabilized on an optimum dosage.

Naltrexone (also an opiate antagonist) used in combination with clonidine hydrochloride (an alpha –2 adrenergic agonist) significantly shortens the period of detoxification from opiates and is probably more effective than methadone detoxification (Charney et al., 1982). However, due to its hypotensive effect, clonidine is usually only used in a hospital setting where the blood pressure can be closely monitored. Lofexidine, which acts in a similar way to clonidine, but has a less sensitive effect on blood pressure, can be used in out-patient opiate detoxification. Naltrexone and Antabuse are commonly used as pharmacological adjuncts in relapse prevention for opiates and alcohol dependency respectively.

In the next section, two case vignettes will be used to illustrate how the particular needs of two polydrug users were met.

Case vignette

Stephen is 25 years old, single and unemployed. At the age of 13, his father was made redundant and the family moved from Scotland to live in a small market town in the south of England, where his father found work in a local factory.. Stephen found it difficult to settle in to his new environment and was teased for his strong Scottish accent. He frequently truanted from school before finally being expelled at the age of 15 for fighting. Over the next five years he smoked cannabis and took amphetamines almost daily, and at weekends took LSD and ecstasy tablets at raves. He was also drinking up to 30 units of alcohol a week.

At this stage, Stephen had left home and rented a room in a house which was also shared by two other drug users. He quickly became immersed into the local drug subculture and got several convictions for shoplifting and burglary to fund his drug and alcohol problem. He was injecting up to four grammes of amphetamines and drinking up to a bottle of spirits daily. In addition he was also injecting temazepam capsules that were either bought illicitly or obtained from various doctors. Stephen was referred to the local community drug and alcohol team by his probation officer following a conviction for shoplifting.

Interventions

Stephen presented in an anxious and agitated state constantly asking for something to calm him down and threatening to leave if he did not receive a prescription of some sort. He had injected amphetamines immediately prior to his appointment with the community psychiatric nurse (CPN) but denied using alcohol or temazepam. Eventually Stephen agreed to complete the interview after being informed that a prescription could only be issued after an assessment was made to determine his medication needs. His physical condition was poor. He had lost nearly two stones in weight over the past couple of months and injecting sites on both his arms appeared infected.

Shortly after his assessment, Stephen was prescribed dexamphetamine elixir and diazepam tablets by his GP on condition that he avoided injecting and kept his appointments with the CPN. Over the next few weeks, his physical and mental state improved, and with the help of the social worker he managed to find new accommodation in a quiet part of town and away from his drug-using peers. In addition to counselling, Stephen attended sessions of anxiety management and later enrolled on a job training scheme as an apprentice mechanic. He was gradually weaned off deaxamphetamines over an eight week period and is currently reducing his diazepam prescription by 5 mg a week.

Case vignette

Jane is 34 years old, single and unemployed. Her parents separated when she was seven and she has not had any contact with her father since. He is said to have been a heavy drinker and violent. Jane finished school at 16 without any qualifications and left home soon afterwards to live with her boyfriend. They both identified with the punk movement of the 1970s and used 'uppers and downers' on a regular basis. Jane drank heavily at the weekends and always to the extent of 'passing out'. The relationship with her boyfriend ended after four years when he left for someone else. This was an extremely painful experience for Jane and it deepened her feelings of rejection. She then became involved with a heroin addict who introduced her to heroin which she began injecting right from the start. She was frequently beaten up by her new boyfriend and on one occasion was hospitalized with a broken jaw. Despite the violence, Jane remained in the relationship for five years during which time she was injecting up to 1g of heroin daily and taking large amounts of benzodiazepines prescribed by her doctor.

Over the next eight years, Jane became more chaotic in her lifestyle, seeking out an existence in bedsitters and acquiring numerous convictions for shoplifting and forging stolen cheques. She was frequently admitted to hospital with drug related complications such as overdoses, abscesses and hepatitis.

Interventions

There were several failed attempts at inpatient detoxification and residential rehabilitation before Jane was eventually stabilized on a prescription of methadone linctus and diazepam. Over a three month period, she stabilized her drug use and received regular counselling as an outpatient. Jane then asked for her methadone to be reduced with a view to coming off altogether as she and her new partner wanted to try for a baby. However, her drinking increased and she began to inject heroin, albeit on a less frequent basis. Shortly afterwards, Jane was admitted to hospital with septicaemia thought to be as a result of unsterile injecting equipment. She became dangerously ill and had to be ventilated for a couple of weeks. She was detoxified from opiates during this period and eventually left hospital with a prescription for 15mg diazepam daily. She is currently living with her mother and attends as an outpatient for weekly counselling and support.

CONCLUSION

The case vignettes cited in this chapter, sketch the development of the typical polydrug using career in two clients and highlight some of the common problems experienced by polydrug users. As a group, they tend to present with complex needs which require a multi-modal approach involving pharmacological, social and psychological interventions. Because polydrug users often lead such chaotic lifestyles, engaging them in a structured therapeutic milieu can be difficult and requires a flexible and client-centred approach from drug workers. This does not necessarily mean acquiescing in requests for medication or tolerating undesirable behaviour, for example turning up intoxicated for appointments or aggressive behaviour. On the other hand, clients should not be expected to attend numerous appointments as part of a lengthy and over cautious assessment procedure before receiving some pharmacological relief for their symptoms. Given the increased risks of HIV infection and overdoses, together with the physical and mental health problems experienced by this cohort of clients, special efforts should be made to remain in contact with them. It is important to establish a trusting therapeutic relationship with the polydrug user, and a sympathetic letter, phone call or community visit may help to re-engage those who have defaulted from treatment.

REFERENCES

Advisory Council on the Misuse of Drugs (1993) *AIDS and Drug Misuse Update: Department of Health*, HMSO, London.

Charney, D.S., Heninger, G.R. and Kleber, H.G. (1982) Clonidine and naltrexone: a safe, effective and rapid treatment of abrupt withdrawal from methadone. *Archives of General Psychiatry*, **39**(3), 1327–32.

Curran, V.H. (1986) Tranquillising memories: a review of the effects of benzodiazepines on human memory. *Biological Psychology*, **23**, 179–213.

Dackis, C.A. and Marks, S.G. (1983) Opiate addiction and depression – cause or effect. *Drug Alcohol Dependence*, **11**(1), 105–9.

Darke, S., Swift, W., Hall, W. and Ross, M. (1993) Drug use, HIV risk-taking and psychosocial correlates of benzodiazepine use among methadone maintenance clients. *Drug and Alcohol Dependence*, **34**(1), 67–70.

Drug Scenes (1987) *A report on drugs and drug dependence by the Royal College of Psychiatrists*, Gaskell, London.

DuPont, R.L. (1988) Abuse of benzodiazepines: The problems and the solutions. *American Journal of Drug and Alcohol Abuse*, **14** (suppl. 1), 1–69.

Frischer, M., Bloor, M., Goldberg, D. *et al.* (1993) Mortality among injecting drug users: A critical re-appraisal. *Journal of Epidemiology Community Health*, **47**(4), 59–63.

Gawin, F.H., Kleber, H.D., Byck, R. *et al.* (1989) Desipramine facilitation of initial cocaine abstinence. *Archives of General Psychiatry*, **46**(2), 117–21.

Ghodse, A.H. (1994) Combined use of drugs and alcohol. *Journal of Current Opinion in Psychiatry*, **7**(3), 249–51.

Hammersley, R., Cassidy, M.T. and Oliver, J. (1995) Drugs associated with drug-related deaths in Edinburgh and Glasgow, November 1990 to October 1992. *Addiction*, **90**(7), 959–65.

Klee, H., Faugier, J., Hayes, C. *et al.* (1990) AIDS-related risk behaviour, polydrug use and temazepam. *British Journal of Addiction*, **85**(19), 1125–32.

Perera, K.M.H., Tulley, M. and Jenner, F.A. (1987) The use of benzodiazepines among drug addicts. *British Journal of Addiction*, **82**(5), 511–15.

Petursson, H. and Lader, M. (1984) *Dependence on Tranquillisers*, Oxford University Press, Oxford.

Ruben, S.M. and Morrison, C.L. (1992) Temazepam misuse in a group of injecting drug users. *British Journal of Addiction*, **87**(10), 1387–92.

Saunders, B., Wilkinson, C. and Phillips, M. (1995) The impact of a brief motivational intervention with opiate users attending a methadone programme. *Addiction*, **90**(3), 415–24.

Schukit, M.A. and Monteiro, M.G. (1988) Alcoholism, anxiety and depression. *British Journal of Addiction*, **83**(12), 1373–80.

<table>
<tr><td>5</td><td># HIV/AIDS and substance misuse: health interventions</td></tr>
</table>

| 5 | # HIV/AIDS and substance misuse: health interventions |

Jan Miller

INTRODUCTION

The advent of HIV and AIDS, in the 1980s, called for a re-examination of substance misuse services. Service provision and interventions were targeted to curb the spread of this new challenge, believed to be a greater danger to individual and public health than drug misuse (ACMD, 1989). The nature of substance misuse problems became an issue at a national policy level, with the emergence of government targets for improved health. These were associated with smoking, alcohol consumption, sharing of injecting equipment and sexual practices, (Health of the Nation, Department of Health, 1992). In 1993, the ACMD recognized the need for improving the efficiency of existing services and interventions through evaluation of targets. Such targets placed an emphasis on the reduction of the extent of drug use with the effect of contributing to HIV prevention.

The aims of this chapter are to address the issues and concerns that substance misuse services have been tackling in order to provide appropriate and effective services. It will also examine the health interventions used to reduce the spread of HIV/AIDS among substance misusers. The first section provides a 'cooks tour' of prevalence of HIV/AIDS and substance misuse and considers the implications for drug and alcohol users in light of prevalence. This is followed by considering the various service strategies and range of interventions necessary to combat the issues, supported by checklists of good practice.

PREVALENCE

The importance of intravenous drug use in the HIV/AIDS epidemic is well recognized, not only through the sharing of injecting equipment, but through sexual contacts. According to the European Centre for the Epidemiological Monitoring of AIDS (1995), nearly two thirds of the AIDS infected population of Spain and Italy acquired their infection through sharing injecting equipment. The proportion of AIDS cases in other European countries who were similarly infected is 39% in Switzerland, 24% in France, 14% in Germany and 6% in the UK.

The level of HIV infection in the UK remains low, with 3% for men and 4% for women in London and the South East and less than 1% in most areas outside London. Prevalence being higher in those who first injected before or during 1985 (Department of Health, 1995a). Data from the unlinked anonymous survey suggest that HIV transmission in injecting drug users has remained low in recent years, despite the sharing of needles by a fifth of injecting drug users and continuing transmission of the hepatitis B virus (Department of Health, 1995a). The higher prevalence of hepatitis B, among injecting drug users, is an indication of involvement in 'risky behaviours', which provides evidence for continued harm reduction efforts. It is projected that, between 1995 and 1999, new AIDS cases will rise by 25% in the heterosexual exposure category and 29% in injecting drug users (PHLS 1996).

MODELS OF HEALTH AND SOCIAL CARE

Although an HIV explosion has not materialized in the UK, to the extent originally feared, injecting drug users remain vulnerable to the risks. This is due to their 'sharing' behaviour, and many are acquiring other blood borne viral infections such as hepatitis B, (Department of Health, 1995). This indicates the continuing need for prevention strategies. The emphasis to 'fine tune' services and interventions is of greater importance today in order to maintain this position. It is essential to avoid complacency, which could give rise to a sudden eruption and rapid spread of disease. Prevention messages and interventions need to be consistently applied not only to the current population of intravenous drug users, but targeted at potential injectors particularly young people – 'drug users on the horizon', since sharing behaviour among younger injectors and women is on the incline (Tackling Drugs Together, 1995).

Service provision and models of intervention in substance misuse, and other areas of health and social care, need to reflect on the considerations raised by the link between drug and alcohol problems and HIV and AIDS. Given that prevalence of HIV and AIDS has not rocketed, services should be organized to ensure effective responses are in place to prevent an explosion and reflect the government's strategy (Tackling Drugs Together, 1995).

It has been suggested that the disinhibiting effects of alcohol can lead to risky sexual behaviour. This, therefore, poses a threat to the general population of a rise in the number of sexually transmitted diseases, including HIV, due to the failure to use condoms (Plant and Plant 1992). Health interventions to address the relationship between alcohol and sexual behaviour need some consideration, if services are to challenge the steady rise in prevalence among the heterosexual population of non-injecting drug users (PHLS, 1996). This is particularly important since alcohol increases the likelihood of sexual activity, with an increased likelihood of sexual risk-taking (Rhodes and Stimson, 1994).

The needs of the population need to be defined in order to create a comprehensive range of appropriate services to meet demands. There should be improving access to specialist inpatient services for detoxification and recovery as well as establishing community services. Addressing the needs of substance misusers requires collaboration across agencies (both statutory and non-statutory) and disciplines to provide a range of effective services and interventions. In response to HIV/AIDS, services should be targeting the whole population from the young to the elderly, with a flexible approach that is easily accessible.

The components of quality service provision should include a variety of options:

- advice, counselling, education and support;
- telephone helpline;
- early intervention services eg. low threshold services, outreach;
- individual treatment packages eg. pharmacotherapeutic interventions, methadone detoxification, longer term methadone treatment, non-opiate detoxification;
- needle and syringe exchange schemes and safe disposal of used equipment;
- HIV counselling and testing;
- health promotion of safer sexual practices.

HIV prevention and outreach

Outreach models were established to bridge the gaps in healthcare provision within the arena of drug misuse, on the premise that those who do not seek help, may be more likely to engage in HIV risk behaviours (Power et al., 1988). The outreach philosophy of 'go out and get them' approach, has become a recognized intervention of reaching out to the hidden populations of drug users, who do not access treatment services (Rhodes, 1993). The main aim of outreach is to offer harm-reduction interventions to hard to reach population groups, eg. information, education and advice, injecting equipment and condoms, in order to reduce the risk of HIV transmission and AIDS. These can be achieved by two complementary broad approaches:

- the initiation of change directly within the community (change in injecting and sexual HIV risk behaviour);
- the initiation of change indirectly, by facilitating the access of individuals, to existing substance misuse services (Rhodes et al., 1991).

A variety of innovative models have been adopted to target those 'at risk', according to the local population. These models include needle and syringe mobile exchange schemes in rural and urban locations, methadone mobile buses (Buning et al., 1990), detached work (working in isolation from established services e.g. 'on the street', in bars, arcades, station concourses and clubs), peripatetic work (working from non-health locations eg. probation offices, prisons, youth centres and other community venues).

Outreach interventions are an integral part of service delivery and should be developed in collaboration with existing services to enhance and develop innovative contacting strategies (ACMD, 1993). It is important to recognize the potential of existing community services to avoid duplication. Individual agencies/ organizations cannot be 'all things to all people', and hence the need to explore the role of the general practitioner for early screening of drug and alcohol problems, general health screening and the provision of family planning. The community pharmacist may also be involved in needle and syringe exchange schemes, advice on local services and health advice (Department of Health, 1996a).

Outreach interventions need to be monitored and evaluated to ensure effectiveness of the strategies employed, according to local needs assessment of the population and existing service provision in order to ensure appropriate targeting.

Appropriate target groups

Appropriate target groups include:

- young people (drug and alcohol users on the horizon);
- women;
- occasional injectors;
- non-opiate users (including cocaine, amphetamine, benzodiazepine and steroid users);
- male and female prostitutes;
- homeless people;
- ethnic/cultural groups;
- those with learning difficulties;
- gay men and lesbians.

Appropriate interventions

Appropriate interventions include:

- distribution of condoms and health education about safer sexual practices;
- distribution of clean injecting equipment and advice on cleaning agents;
- advice on the risks of sharing and educational 'use your own' messages;
- community based drop-in centres in appropriate locations;
- community drop-in centres in primary healthcare settings;
- satellite HIV testing and HIV counselling facilities;
- needle and syringe exchange schemes via community pharmacies.

HIV pre- and post-test counselling

Advice, education and counselling on HIV should now be part of mainstream clinical care (Department of Health, 1996b), particularly within the field of substance misuse, due to the obvious risks. Although HIV testing is not a compulsory condition of treatment, clients at high risk (those who share injecting equipment and those at risk due to their sexual behaviour) should be encouraged to consider having a test (Ghodse 1995) as there are possible clinical benefits of early diagnosis of HIV (ACMD, 1995). Staff need to have appropriate experience, skills and training to undertake HIV pre- and post-test counselling. Also they need to ensure that they are aware of current developments in the management of HIV and AIDS.

Pre-test counselling

The main aim of pre-test counselling is to provide the patient/client with the opportunity to understand the implications of either a negative or positive test. This should be discussed within the context of their injecting and sexual risk behaviours and they should be prepared so that they can make informed choices. All workers should be equipped with the skills and knowledge to undertake assessment of HIV risk behaviours and provide harm-reduction advice. Although, the specialist pre- and post-test counselling, may well be conducted by those staff who receive specialist training, it is important to recognize that allocation of time to undertake pre- and post-test counselling will need to reflect the individual needs of the patient. In a study undertaken by the (Department of Health, 1996b), the longest average length of counselling session was undertaken by Drug Dependency Clinics (31–60 minutes), while GPs spent the shortest (0–10 minutes).

It is crucial that the individual undertaking the pre-test counselling understands the implications for themselves, in the context of health, social, psychological, financial and legal issues. To ensure a consistent approach among staff, it is good practice to have policy and practice guidelines in all substance misuse services, in line with national guidelines.

Pre-test discussion
This includes the implications of testing:

- education on viral transmission, the manifestations of the HIV virus and the nature of the test and the difference between HIV and AIDS;
- assessment of perceived and actual risk behaviours and education on risk reduction;
- discussion on the implications of both a negative and a positive test result, including seroconversion, the impact on family and partner(s), pregnancy, the limitations of the test (does not identify time of transmission or predict the future course of events), psychological impact, life insurance, mortgages, employment;
- information about the confidentiality policy. All services offering a testing facility need to have confidentiality policies regarding the disclosure of test results, recording and storage of results. This is particularly important when client

records are held centrally in an organization and accessible to other services e.g. mental health teams. Clients need to be aware that within statutory services, information may be shared with other members of the team including the client's GP. It is important to explore any concerns regarding confidentiality with the patient and explain the importance of the GP as primary carer, having knowledge of treatment and tests undertaken by the specialist services;

- information regarding time scale for receiving the results and how they will be given;
- patients should be advised about cleaning blood spillages, be warned about the risks of sharing toothbrushes and razors (which may come into contact with blood) and also be informed about preventative measures against hepatitis B and C;
- the patient must be given the opportunity to have time to think about the issues before making a decision.

The pre-test checklist is given in Table 5.1.

Post-test counselling

The result of the HIV test should be given to the patient face to face, preferably by the pre-test counsellor. It is not advisable to give results over the telephone or by writing as responses are difficult to assess. More importantly, if there is a lack of consistency across services, a patient may wrongly presume a positive test result if a counsellor requests a face to face contact, when the patient has previously experienced results being given over the telephone. Staff should avoid giving results (particularly a positive test result) at the last appointment of the day or before going on leave, to ensure their availability for the patient to have further discussions. The post-test discussion checklist is given in Table 5.2.

It is not uncommon for patients to perceive that they are immune, when they have exposed themselves to risks and receive a negative test result, and to assume that they do not need to change their behaviour. The use of analogies to explain such events can be useful in assisting the individual to take continued responsibility

Table 5.1 Pre-test checklist

- Ensure the individual understands the nature of HIV infection, provision of information about HIV transmission and risk reduction
- Discuss at risk activities in which the individual may have been involved with respect to HIV infection including the date of the last risk activity and the perception of the need for the test
- Provision of written information
- Discuss the benefits and difficulties to the individual, his or her family and associates of having a test and knowing the result whether positive or negative
- Provide details of the test and how the result will be provided
- Obtain an informed decision about whether or not to proceed with the test

Table 5.2 Post-test checklist

- Address immediate concerns and provide support to those who are positive
- Re-emphasize information on prevention of HIV transmission whether the test is negative or positive

If the test result is positive

- Address the patient's immediate reaction
- Refer to specialist management, including treatment where appropriate
- Provide details of local support services and national organizations eg. Terrence Higgins Trust and Body Positive
- Offer follow up counselling and ongoing support, which may include repeating information which may have been forgotten and addressing issues concerned with legal matters, how to inform family and other associates, support for carers and partner(s) and testing for associates

---

for their behaviour, for example, someone who crosses the road several times a day is more likely to be knocked over than someone who crosses the road once a week, likewise with risky behaviours.

It is necessary to ensure that there are collaborative working arrangements and policies regarding liaison with relevant appropriate services eg. genitourinary medicine (GUM), communicable diseases units, specialist HIV/AIDS services and voluntary organizations such as buddy schemes. The emotional and psychological impact of undertaking HIV counselling, can be difficult for the counsellor, and must not be underestimated. This emphasizes the importance of the need for appropriate access to clinical supervision and support.

Models of service provision for pre- and post-test counselling and testing facilities

Those who wish to have an HIV antibody test should be able to do so with the minimum of inconvenience, (Department of Health, 1996b) and therefore services need to develop pre- and post-test counselling and testing arrangements according to local service provision, geographical service location and accessibility, availability of trained staff and allocation of resources. It may be appropriate in some areas to have joint working arrangements with local services eg. GUM clinics or GPs.

The possible models for consideration are:

1. Full in-house service, which provides the full service on site by the substance misuse service, including, pre- and post-test counselling and testing by trained staff within the substance misuse service.
2. On-site service for counselling, testing provided by an outside service, whereby pre- and post-test counselling is provided by the substance misuse team but the patient is then referred to other services for blood taking eg. the local hospital or GP.

3. Outside service providing pre- and post-test counselling, testing provided by an outside service, whereby pre and post-test counselling is provided on site in the substance misuse service, by an outside agency e.g. a visiting counsellor, who may have responsibility for more than one service area. Patients are also referred to an outside service eg. the local hospital or to the GP, for venepuncture.

4. Referral to other services for access to counselling and screening. Pre- and post-test counselling is referred to other local services eg. local statutory substance misuse service, GUM clinic or GP. This arrangement may be more favoured by non-statutory drug and/or alcohol agencies (who may not have access to staff trained to provide venepuncture facilities), rural satellite clinics, hostels or residential rehabilitation units.

These models can be adapted to meet the health needs of the population, the substance misuse service and local resources to ensure effective, accessible and flexible service provision without duplicating services. Although it may be more cost effective to refer patients to outside services, where counselling and testing are provided already, it is important to monitor the uptake of the service to determine the most appropriate model of service provision. Substance misuse services may find that offering on site services increases uptake by capitalizing on opportunistic access.

Case vignette

Mary aged 35 years was brought to a drop-in low threshold clinic by a friend. She had never approached drug services previously despite her 15-year history of drug misuse and prostitution. During the initial assessment, she admitted to sharing needles and syringes and not using condoms with her clients in order to obtain more money to fund her heroin habit. On examination, there were obvious signs of injecting (track) marks and abscesses on her thighs as a result of injecting into her groins. A urine analysis resulted in the positive identification of opiate and it was decided to prescribe oral methadone mixture to engage her in order to address her health and social problems in particular her high risk behaviours. Further intervention strategies included, in the short-term, liaison with her GP and local hospital for her physical problems, exploration of her drug misuse and her status regarding HIV and hepatitis, perception of risks behaviours, and health education and harm-minimization in terms of safer sex and safer drug use. On a medium- to long-term, Mary would be engaged in the management of her drug use and assisted to making changes in her lifestyle.

NURSING INTERVENTIONS

Nurses working in all areas of healthcare need to be familiar with issues of both substance misuse and HIV/AIDS. It should be recognized that both infection and non-infection related to HIV medical conditions can mimic medical conditions associated with injecting drug use, nurses need to be familiar with the issues related to both substance misuse and HIV/AIDS, (Brettle, 1996). This is particularly important in the primary healthcare setting, where patients are more likely to ask for advice on physical health. It is crucial therefore that primary healthcare nurses are equipped to be able to screen and assess substance use and misuse at an early stage.

Nurses can easily identify a specific health promotional role in reducing the spread of hepatitis and HIV/AIDS, through educating patients about their risk behaviours and empowering them to take an active part in changing behaviour. Nurses are often on the front line and therefore in a prime position to assess risk behaviours, including the sharing of injecting equipment (needles, syringes, spoons and filters) and unprotected sexual practices. It is useful to explore with the patient, whether they understand the risks of their behaviour, whether it is viewed as an occupational hazard, or how they perceive their risk-taking. It must never be presumed that patients are knowledgable about the health hazards of their substance use. They may be embarrassed to admit sharing injecting equipment or unsafe/disinhibited sexual practices, or may deny their actual behaviours or lack of knowledge, for fear of being judged by professionals.

Nurses can make a significant contribution as health educators by providing patients, as well as other nursing colleagues, with education and information about health issues related to substance misuse. Clients and carers affected by hepatitis and HIV or AIDS require ongoing support in coping with the consequences of their drug and/or alcohol use. Nurses can focus on these emotional and psychological needs by providing supportive counselling to facilitate the patient's feelings and acceptance or denial of their condition. Nurses have a clear role in acting as health promotors, educators, counsellors/therapists within the multidisciplinary team in preventative work. They also provide a holistic approach to care as well as acting as a link to other professionals and coordinator of care, as required (e.g. HIV services, hepatologists).

CONCLUSION

The message is clear. HIV and AIDS are here to stay and how services choose to respond with regard to substance use and misuse, will depend on the effectiveness of tackling the issues to prevent an HIV/AIDS boom. No one approach or service can provide services effectively to the total population and there is, therefore, the need for collaboration across all agencies and disciplines.

The focus of development for the 90s and moving into the 21st century is to continue to prevent HIV and AIDS through monitoring and evaluating existing and new services/interventions to meet the changing needs. With the move to a primary care led health service, the impetus has evolved to share the responsibility with primary healthcare services, (Department of Health, 1995b). Such developments have an impact on the specialist services in formulating agreements regarding prevention, care and treatment and continuing care. Greater emphasis needs to be placed on understanding the behaviours associated with sexual and injecting risk behaviours in order to have an impact on facilitating change.

REFERENCES

ACMD (1989) *AIDS and Drug Misuse, part 2*. Report by the Advisory Council on the Misuse of Drugs, HMSO, London.

ACMD (1995) *AIDS and Drug Misuse Update*. Report by the Advisory Council on the Misuse of Drugs, HMSO, London.

Brettle, R.P. (1996) Clinical features of drug use and drug use related HIV, Editorial Review, *International Journal of STD & AIDS*, **7**(3), 151–65.

Buning, E., Van Brussel, G. and Van Santen, G. (1990) The 'methadone by bus project' in Amsterdam. *British Journal of Addiction*, **85**(10), 1247–50.

Department of Health (1992) *Health of the Nation: A Strategy for Health in England*, HMSO, London.

Department of Health (1995a) Unlinked Anonymous HIV Surveys Steering Group, Public Health Laboratory Service (PHLS), The Institute of Child Health, University of London. *Unlinked anonymous HIV seroprevalence monitoring programme in England and Wales – data to the end of 1994*. Department of Health, London.

Department of Health (1995b) Reviewing shared care arrangements for drug misusers. *EL* (95) 114

Department of Health (1996a) *Task Force to review services for Drug Misuse*, Department of Health, London.

Department of Health (1996b) *Guidelines for pre-test discussion on HIV testing*, Department of Health, Leeds.

European Centre for the Epidemiological Monitoring of AIDS (1995) HIV/AIDS Surveillance in Europe. *Quarterly Report, No. 48*.

Ghodse, A.H. (1995) *Drugs and Addictive Behaviour – A Guide to Treatment*, 2nd edn, Blackwell Science, Oxford.

Power, R., Hartnoll, R. and Daviaud, E. (1988) Drug injecting, AIDS and risk behaviour: potential for change and intervention strategies. *British Journal of Addiction*, **83**(b), 649–54.

PHLS (1996) *Communicable Diseases Report. The incidence and prevalence of AIDS and prevalence of other severe HIV disease in England and Wales for 1995 to 1999: projections using data to the end of 1994*, **6**(1), No. 1, January.

Plant, M.L & Plant, M A (1992) *Risk Takers*, London, Routledge.

Rhodes, T., Holland, J., Hartnoll, R., and Johnson, A. (1991) *HIV Outreach Health Education: National and International Perspectives. Summary Report to the Department of Health, Drug Indicators Project*, University of London.

Rhodes, T. (1993) Time for community change:what has outreach to offer? Editorial, *Addiction*, **88**(11), 1553–60.

Rhodes, T. and Stimson, G.V. (1994) What is the relationship between drug taking and sexual risk? Social relations and social research. *Sociology of Health and Illness*, **16**(2), 209–28.

Tackling Drugs Together: A strategy for England 1995–98 (1995), HMSO, London.

Alcohol and alcohol problems: nursing interventions | 6

David Cooper

INTRODUCTION

Alcohol and alcohol-related problems play an important role in nurses' day-to-day client contact. Some alcohol related problems and the required nursing interventions are clear, for example, clinical supervision during alcohol withdrawal, intensive care following alcohol overdose or a calm considered approach during an aggressive outburst from a problem drinker. Others are not so evident. For example, the leg wound that fails to heal because alcohol is affecting the body's natural healing potential, the individual who attends with a work related injury, the distressed mother who complains that her baby constantly cries, and who, on closer assessment, is found to have a problem drinking partner. The anxieties associated with financial difficulties are exhibited through the child. Thus, all professional nursing groups have an obligation to assess for alcohol use and misuse.

This chapter presents a brief overview of the nature and extent of problem drinking and drinking problems and the nursing interventions required. In particular, an introduction to community alcohol detoxification is presented, and the concept of controlled drinking is examined.

NATURE AND EXTENT OF PROBLEM DRINKING AND DRINKING PROBLEMS

Alcohol use and misuse have a major impact on society. As our society's favoured drug, it plays an integral role in our daily lives. Statistics related to alcohol consumption and the effects on society reveal the extent of the problem. It is suggested that 85% of crime in pubs and clubs and 50% of street crime occur while the offender is intoxicated. In 1992, 69 000 people were cautioned or found guilty of being drunk and disorderly in a public place. For the employer, workplace studies suggest that 75% of employers feel that alcohol misuse is a problem in their organization with an estimated 8.14 million days lost per annum resultant from alcohol related problems (Alcohol Concern, 1995). Alcohol misuse has a noticeable effect on the family and is a key factor in 20% of child abuse cases. 30% of individuals receiving treatment identified alcohol as a major problem in marital conflict. In terms of cost to the nation's health, the NHS spends £150 million per annum on alcohol related problems (Alcohol Concern, 1995).

The consequences of the use and misuse of alcohol can be seen in addiction nurses' regular client contact. The individual does not have to drink at harmful levels to experience, either directly or as a victim, the consequences of inappropriate use i.e. drink driving, work related accidents, sporting accident, aggression, etc. In addition many drug misusers also misuse alcohol.

COMMUNITY DETOXIFICATION

Stockwell (1987) defined detoxification as 'a treatment designed to control both medical and psychological complications that may occur temporarily after a period of heavy and sustained alcohol use'. Most individuals withdrawing from alcohol do not require medication or intensive supervision. However, those who do require clinically supervised intervention should receive care in an effective, safe and humane manner. Admission to hospital during alcohol withdrawal is rarely indicated. It has been suggested that many admissions are ineffective and inappropriate, often failing to meet the needs of the problem drinker, and with re-admission rates as high as 73% (Cooper, 1994a). The problem drinker is often reluctant to seek therapeutic intervention because of stigma and labelling. Such problems are particularly acute in women, who form 30% of the community detoxification client group (Cooper, 1985; Alcohol Research Group (ARG), 1993), and additional resources, support and childcare considerations are often identified as a prerequisite to seeking help.

Concern for the problem drinker provoked a predominantly nursing led intervention referred to as community, or home, detoxification. It is now generally accepted that problem drinkers respond well to inexpensive, minimal interventions. It has been suggested that community detoxification is more effective with problem drinkers who had remained abstinent for a substantial period of time in the past. Those who do return to drinking tend to do so in a more controlled and less harmful manner (ARG, 1993).

Community assessment and detoxification have many advantages for the problem drinker, the family and health purchasers and providers, both from a cost effective and client satisfaction perspective (Table 6.1). As a structured procedure, community detoxification requires a mutual partnership between the nurse, the client and the family. The problem drinker can access family and other existing support networks, while feeling secure in the home environment. However, there is a need for vigilant screening for suitability and those who require clinically supervised detoxification will need close monitoring.

Table 6.1 Advantages of assessment and community detoxification

Decrease in:	Stigma and labelling
	Self discharge
	Time off work
	Work related problems, e.g. accidents, absenteeism
Increase in:	Completion of treatment
	Maintained client access
	Family support
	Self and medical practitioner referral
	Access to women (30% client group)
Assessment:	With full assessment, procedure is safe
	Decreased in-patient care and bed occupancy
	Rules out intensive, inappropriate treatment at home
	Uses existing support network
	Ensure treatment is specific to client needs
	Aids family support at a crucial time

Community detoxification should not be considered as a 'catch all' solution to alcohol withdrawal. It is not suitable or appropriate for everyone withdrawing from alcohol. Stockwell (1987) suggests that assessment to establish the suitability and need for a supervised community detoxification should address two specific questions:

1. Is there a need for any medication to cover withdrawal symptoms?
2. Are there any reasons for not keeping the client within the home environment for detoxification?

The disadvantages of community detoxification should be fully assessed. The home environment may contain excessive triggers that would rule against community detoxification: For example:

- regular alcohol consumption at home;
- easy access to alcohol;
- lack of family support;
- other family member(s) with drinking problem;
- medication used during detoxification.

A primary function of the nurse supervising community detoxification is the monitoring of prescribed medication used to control withdrawal symptoms and its interaction with other substances. Any prescribed medication should be limited and specific – given over an agreed duration in a reducing dosage. Drugs used include chlordiazepoxide and diazepam. It has been suggested that as many as 60% of problem drinkers are vitamin deficient and will require high potency vitamin therapy (Majundar et al., 1981; Editorial: Lancet 1979). Vitamins B1 (thiamine), B6 (pyridoxine) and C (ascorbic acid), are important nutrients normally deficient in problem drinkers, therefore it is advisable to administer vitamin replacement prophylactically.

Alcohol detoxification is merely part of the overall treatment. It is not a prerequisite to every treatment intervention. Therapeutic intervention commences immediately contact is made with the client. However, it is one in which the nurse plays a key role and that will place many demands on their individual skills and expertise. Whether the client requires supervised withdrawal, hospital admission, education and advice can be identified by an eclectic and holistic assessment process which should continue throughout client contact if interventions are to be effective.

Controlled drinking

Davies (1962), noted that when following-up a group of individuals diagnosed as 'alcoholic' that some appeared to be drinking 'normally'. This figure was suggested to be as high as 20%. Soon, other professionals, having experienced similar findings, began to look closer at the concept of harm free drinking and controlled drinking (Heather and Robertson, 1983). Strategies designed to develop self monitoring techniques using a drinking diary have proved to be effective and, as such, have opened other 'options' for the problem drinker. Controlled drinking involves the relearning of drinking habits and behaviour, and this need to relearn drinking behaviour distinguishes the controlled drinker from the 'normal drinker.' The task is not easy and therefore is not appropriate for all individuals. However, it is an option that has met with client approval in that the changes required:

- offer an alternative to abstinence;
- the impact on lifestyle and leisure activity is less dramatic;
- the reduction in intake is reflective of normal drinking behaviour;
- offer some acceptance criteria for controlled drinking programmes (Table 6.2).

Table 6.2 Criteria for controlled drinking

Clients should:

- Choose the controlled drinking goal;
- Be prepared for a brief (3–6 months) period of abstinence prior to commencing programme;
- Be able to recount past safer, social drinking events;
- Not be severely dependent on alcohol (assessment tools, i.e. SADQ will assist in decision-making process);
- Have no evidence of long-term liver damage/seizures/DTs;
- Show no evidence of intellectual/memory impairment;
- Have spouse/friend/partner who agrees to non-abstinence goal (essential).

The difference between normal drinking behaviour (i.e. normal as is currently acceptable by society) and controlled drinking is best described in the following way. The normal drinker drinks on occasions, is clear in his or her ability to be able to exercise choice relating to consumption, and at a point can cease consumption. This does not involve any deliberate decision on behalf of the drinker. The decision to avoid difficulty relating to excessive consumption is taken quickly and effectively without turmoil. The controlled drinker is less confident in his or her drinking. Past experiences have left the individual insecure and acutely aware of the consequences of any laps in concentration. Thus, the controlled drinker needs to be constantly vigilant, choosing with care the occasion, time, place, circumstance and planned limit of consumption. This involves a considerable amount of careful and often compulsive planning prior to any drinking occasion.

The controlled drinker can best be described as an individual who has significant experience of problems in life associated with excessive alcohol consumption. There is a need to recognize that they need to exercise a greater degree of control over their drinking behaviour. Having selected the middle course, between abstinence and uncontrolled consumption, the person has made the choice to set appropriate restrictions on his or her level of alcohol consumption.

Once the individual has learnt to be vigilant, and apply methods of self control over alcohol consumption, the individual has applied these methods effectively and found them to be effective and appropriate for his or her needs.

Assessment

An holistic and eclectic assessment is the key to effective therapeutic intervention. Assessment should not be considered to be a one off exercise but as an ongoing process to ensure that appropriate changes or modifications can be initiated as required. Assessment of alcohol related problems should include the following areas:

- drinking profile – include current use/misuse, client and family opinion and history;
- physical and/or psychological complaints or effects;
- marital and social consequences;.
- employment – status and effect;
- housing and associated problems;
- financial difficulties;
- use and misuse of other substances;
- previous interventions and agencies involved;
- criminal behaviour;
- physical examination including blood pressure and tests, pulse and temperature, breathalyser;
- home environment assessment.

Screening tools

There are several screening tools the nurse can use to assist in assessment for need, suitability and monitoring of detoxification. These include:

- severity of alcohol dependence questionnaire (SADQ) (Stockwell *et al.*, 1983);
- problems inventory (PI) (Stockwell *et al.*, 1983);
- Home environment assessment (HEA) (Bennie, 1991);
- Symptom severity checklist (Murphy *et al.*, 1983).

There are many screening tools and their choice of preference often depends on personal preference. They assist the nurse to assess the level of dependence and depth of support the client and family will need during alcohol detoxification. However, one should be aware that such tools do not make one an 'expert' and are not substitutes for sound clinical judgement. Liver function tests and full blood count should also form part of the assessment and ongoing monitoring. A full and detailed assessment ensures that whichever intervention is chosen, the procedure will be safe and meeting needs. It prevents the need for inappropriate admissions or inappropriate intensive home detoxification. Such assessment will provide the nurse with clearly defined needs and facilitate access to appropriate support networks and specifically designed treatment packages.

NURSING INTERVENTIONS

Nurses play a vital role, not only in the treatment of those who experience alcohol related problems, but in the early identification and intervention of drinking problems. It has been suggested (Cooper, 1994b) that all nurses should be trained to:

- identify the individual with a substance related problem;
- recognize the types of problems likely to be experienced by the individual;
- assist the individual in the process of acknowledging, exploring and understanding the substance related problem;
- appreciate the individual's own perception of the problem;
- consider with the individual the treatment options available;
- facilitate the individual's achievement of the chosen goal(s);
- introduce the individual to services and facilities available to assist;
- act in a nonjudgmental way;
- provide nursing interventions in withdrawal;
- provide support and understanding should relapse occur.

Offering appropriate levels of intervention and support, subsequent to thorough assessment, is an integral part of the nurse's role, the nature and extent of which is dependent on the identified needs of the individual.

The following case vignettes highlight the effectiveness of nursing intervention on two levels. Case 1 involved brief educational intervention and case 2 involves the skills in the identification of a problem, effective liaison and communication with the client and other agencies (primarily the GP), clinical skills in the monitoring of home detoxification, and interpretation of clinical information received through ongoing assessment.

Case Vignette

Colin was a 23-year-old salesman whose hobbies included jogging. He had participated in many local 'fun runs' raising funds for charities and having a keen competitive nature, liked to train hard and often. He would run 10 miles in the morning and a further 10 miles after work. For the past two months or so, Colin had noticed that completing the 20 miles daily jog was proving to be a problem. Initially, he had put this down to a chill, especially as his chest became painful and he often felt excessively breathless and light headed. He had had several minor stumbles during training but none quite as bad as the one that brought him to the accident and emergency department that evening. Colin has fallen on the final part of his run and twisted his ankle.

The A and E triage nurse routinely included questions relating to alcohol consumption in her assessment procedure. On talking to Colin she became concerned about his level of alcohol use. Colin's sales job included many business lunches and social business meetings which involved alcohol consumption. He also likes the occasional pint and would stop every evening on completion of his run to visit the local pub. Recently, this has involved a consumption level of up to 15 standards drinks per day.

The nurse was able to discuss the effects of his alcohol consumption and gave him simple advice on sensible drinking, a drinking diary and information about the general effects of heavy alcohol use. It became clear that while Colin was not dependent on alcohol, he was unaware of his levels of consumption and the effects this was having on his health. This brief intervention was all that was required by this client. Such forms of brief intervention are suggested to lead to significant changes in drinking behaviour (Watson, 1992).

Case Vignette

Mary drinks throughout the day between half to a full bottle of sherry or occasionally cider. Since her children have grown up and left home, she had more time, which she found hard to fill. Her partner, a busy company director, had initially been sympathetic towards her drinking, but was becoming less tolerant, having had to miss several important meetings because of his wife's distressed telephone calls to him while drunk.

Mary visited her GP complaining of insomnia and, during the discussion her level of alcohol consumption was raised. Mary's GP referred her to the community alcohol team and, on assessment, it was agreed that she should be considered for community detoxification. Further assessment revealed that Mary has always liked a drink, but over the last two years had been unable at times to control her consumption. It was noted that Mary's alcohol consumption increased within the week preceding menstruation and she felt it helped her 'feel better'. This 'urge' had occurred about the same time that Mary had decided to stop her hormone replacement therapy (HRT) because of the recent scares discussed on television.

Mary successfully completed her home detoxification and continues to receive ongoing support from the community nurse. She attends the women's group held at the alcohol treatment unit twice a week. Her fears relating to HRT were discussed with the GP who referred Mary back to the consultant responsible for her care. Mary has now recommenced her HRT programme and feels more content with this. At present she is not craving for alcohol and is currently looking at ways in which she can play an active role in her community to fill the vacuum left by her children's departure. There are still a considerable number of steps to take but the outlook is looking better for Mary.

In this study the nurse's expertise and interpretation of the ongoing assessment data helped her to develop a clearer picture of the link between the alcohol use and a physical health problem requiring medical intervention. Her daily support and clinical monitoring of the alcohol withdrawal ensured a safe environment while facilitating much needed support and active intervention.

Brief intervention

Nursing interventions and the level at which such interventions take place vary. Primarily the emphasis of such brief intervention is earlier rather than later, and consist of simple advice and exchange of information which has proved to be effective in influencing a change in drinking behaviour (Watson, 1992). Prochaska and DiClemente (1986), suggest that problem drinking is likely to decrease or be modified to less harmful levels at a point of change. These changes include life events such as childbirth, marriage or crises, such as accident or hospital admission. Cooper (1995) offers some practical advice on brief intervention.

1. When drinking is not seen as a problem: the best course of action is one of education and harm-minimization. Offering low key verbal and written advice is essential education. By providing simple written material the individual is given the opportunity to return to this later.
2. If alcohol is acknowledged as a problem but help seeking is not yet being considered: offer verbal and written advice plus details of support and advisory services. Offer to facilitate contact with the support and advisory agencies if required.
3. Harmful consumption is not seen as a problem and the individual does not request help: offer advice within the individual limitations, and contact details of helping agencies. Offer to initiate contact with support and advisory agencies.
4. Wants to cease consumption or modify drinking behaviour and may require clinically supervised withdrawal: make contact with alcohol advisory service for further advice and guidance.

The depth and extent of nursing interventions vary depending on the level of skill and experience of the nurse providing such intervention. The above list outlines four differing levels of intervention in which the nurse plays a key role. The list is not exhaustive.

CONCLUSION

Nurses are active in statutory and voluntary sector services at prevention, intervention and treatment levels. Such services include alcohol advisory services and alcohol treatment units participating in structured residential programmes. Others work in predominantly nurse led projects such as the Turning Point initiative in Manchester (Smithfield project) where anyone requiring detoxification can walk in at any time, in any state of intoxication and is accepted provided there is a bed available. Such projects have met with a great deal of success and are to be commended.

The level of involvement depends on the nurses' expertise and includes counselling, psychotherapy, family therapy, education and training. The nurse has many skills to offer the problem drinking client and those experiencing drinking problems. Many new initiatives in care are nurse led often out of necessity, but they are considerably effective. It is essential however, that all nurses should consider identification and intervention in problem drinking behaviour as an integral part of their role.

REFERENCES

Alcohol Concern (1995) *What about alcohol?* (An alcohol education pack), Alcohol Concern, London.

Alcohol Research Group (1993) *Home detoxification for problem drinkers: a pilot study*, Alcohol Research Group, Edinburgh University, Report on the 15th year, pp. 5–6.

Bennie, C. (1991) *Home detoxification service for problem drinkers*. Report for 4th Valley Health Authority, Scotland. Personal Communication.

Cooper, D.B. (1985) *The effects of a community alcohol service, the hidden 'potential drinking problems' and problem drinking*. Report to the District Management Team, Blackburn, Hyndburn and Ribble Valley Health Authority.

Cooper, D.B. (1994a) *Alcohol Home Detoxification and Assessment*, Radcliffe Medical Press, Oxford.

Cooper, D.B. (1994b) The person with dependency problems, in *Nursing practice: hospital and home – the adult* (eds M.F. Alexander, J.N. Fawcett and P.J. Runciman), Churchill Livingstone, Edinburgh.

Cooper, D.B. (1995) Habit-forming questions. *Nursing Times*, **91**(44), 36–7.

Davies, X. (1962) Normal drinking in recovered alcohol addicts. *Quarterly Journal of Studies on Alcohol*, **23**, 94–104.

Editorial (1979) Wernicker's preventable encephalopathy. *Lancet*, I, 1122–3.

Heather, N. and Robertson, I. (1983) *Controlled Drinking*, Cambridge University Press, Cambridge.

Leading Article (1979) *British Medical Journal*, **21**(6185), 291–2.

Majundar, S.K., Shaw, G.K. and Thomson, A.D. (1981). Blood vitamin status in chronic alcoholics after a single dose of polyvitamin: a preliminary report. *Postgraduate Medical Journal*, **57**, 164–6.

Murphy, D.J., Shaw, G.K. and Clark, I. (1983) Tiapride and chlormethiazole in alcohol withdrawal: a double blind trial. *Alcohol and Alcoholism*, **18**(3), 227–37.

Prochaska, J.O. and DiClemente, C.C. (1986) *Towards a comprehensive model of change, in treating addictive behaviours: process of change* (eds W.R. Miller and N. Heather), Plenum, London.

Stockwell, T. (1987) The Exeter home detoxification project, in *Helping the problem drinker: a new initiative in community care* (eds T. Stockwell and S. Clement), Croom Helm, London.

Stockwell, T., Murphy, D.J. and Hodgson, R. (1983) The severity of alcohol dependence questionnaire: its reliability and validity. *British Journal of Addiction*, **78**(2), 145–55.

Watson, H.E. (1992) A study of the effectiveness of brief intervention for problem drinkers in acute hospital setting. University of Strathclyde, Glasgow. Dissertation.

Relapse prevention and nursing interventions

7

Claudia Salazar

INTRODUCTION

Relapse prevention (RP) offers a comprehensive theory for specialist nurses working in the drug and alcohol field that can be effectively applied, particularly in the community health setting. When attempting to offer ongoing support following an initial period of treatment this often involves the management of relapse. RP acknowledges the biological, psychological and sociocultural factors involved in addictive behaviours. Thus, it values a wide range of relapse management strategies from the use of disulfiram to the use of the AA fellowship. The high relapse rate over time, following treatment for addictive behaviours has long been recognized. Addressing the factors involved in the relapse process has led to the acknowledgement of the real difficulties that individuals have to encounter when trying to achieve a substance-free lifestyle. RP incorporates work on motivation and motivational interviewing (Miller, 1983; Miller 1985) and the model of change (Prochaska and DiClemente, 1982).

The aim of this chapter is to provide a brief overview of the RP model involving the process of change. The importance of a treatment matching approach and implications for nursing practice will be addressed. The chapter will also describe the process of setting up a RP group for problem drinkers.

MOTIVATION AND STAGES OF CHANGE

Traditional approaches tend to view motivation as a personal trait or state which is shown by the use of defense mechanisms such as 'denial' by the client. These are interpreted as being part of the personality of the 'alcoholic' that is a barrier to treatment. However, research has shown that there is no evidence for 'addictive personality' types and that motivation for treatment is greatly influenced by the interaction between client and therapist (Miller, 1985). Thus, confrontation generally elicits a defensive stance on the part of the client and that more empathic counselling styles can be more successful. A model of change was first described by Prochaska and DiClemente (1982) as a result of their study of smokers who were successful in quitting. They found that change occurred in a series of steps. In a recent paper, Prochaska, DiClemente and Norcross 1992) summarize the research on the basic constructs of the model and have revised this linear progression. They have now described a 'spiral model of change' acknowledging that most people will relapse but do not regress to the point where they began. This means that relapse does not involve an endless 'revolving door' process but that they learn from their mistakes and move forward.

Motivational interviewing is a counselling approach which aims to facilitate and engage clients in the process of change. It aims to raise awareness and enhance decision-making, and it is at its most valuable when clients are in the pre-contemplation and contemplation stage (Miller, 1985). In particular, when working with problem drinkers, motivational interviewing offers a way of approaching the initial interview with a client. It shows how to assess their perception of the situation and therefore enables nurses to target their intervention depending on the assessment of the stage of change. This is particularly important for nurses working in a nonspecialist setting, usually in a liaison function such as in general practice or general hospital departments, when clients are more likely to have little or no awareness of the effects of their alcohol intake.

TREATMENT MATCHING

There is common acknowledgement that there is not one superior treatment modality that is effective for all individuals experiencing an alcohol problem, and that there are complex variables for each individual (Miller, 1985, 1989; Lindstrom, 1992). Therefore the treatment matching hypothesis implies that if an individual is matched to a particular treatment according to certain criteria the outcome will be improved. This implies that a systematized sequence of decisions involved in assessment treatment and follow-up is required to maximize the outcome for any individual.

The implications of treatment matching are that it enables nurses to systematize their assessment and case management process and to begin to establish criteria for the treatment options recommended to clients based on shared principles. Although criteria for treatment matching are not clear, some factors that are highlighted in the available literature are reflected by current clinical practice in the community. The components of a comprehensive nursing assessment need to reflect the importance of establishing individual treatment plans based on the degree of vulnerability that will dictate the intensity of intervention needed. A comprehensive assessment in the community can take up to three sessions, and may require involvement from other members of the multidisciplinary team. Objective tools that can confirm clinical judgement such as questionnaires should be considered as well as routine blood tests. Unless the individual is in crisis, time needs to be spent in developing a rapport with the client as well as enhancing motivation and decision-making. The treatment options should be discussed from a multidisciplinary perspective. Specialist nurses in the community have the function of enabling clients to access the right treatment agency based on careful assessment and with the full involvement of clients and their families or significant others. Nurses can advise and enable clients to access the most appropriate treatment option as well as offering ongoing support, evaluation and follow-up.

WHAT IS RELAPSE PREVENTION?

RP is a model of understanding the relapse process and was first outlined by Alan Marlatt (1979). This is based on social learning theory of behaviour change (Bandura, 1977) and differs radically from previous models of addictive behaviours, such as the disease model. Table 7.1 highlights the differences between the two models.

With the introduction of RP there was the development of a variety of cognitive behavioural approaches in the treatment of addictive behaviours. Some have concentrated on self-efficacy (Annis and Davis, 1987), adapted to the 12 step treatment approach (Gorski, 1986; 1990), and used in conjunction with pharmacological treatments (Annis and Peachey, 1992) as well as with cue exposure (Hodgson and Rankin, 1982). Although the effectiveness of RP compared to traditional hospital treatment has been demonstrated (Allsop and Saunders, 1989), the methodological difficulties involved in comparing one treatment approach to another, and the lack of controlled trials makes it difficult to decide on the relative effectiveness

Table 7.1 Difference between relapse prevention and disease model

Relapse prevention		Disease model
Education approach which fosters detachment of self from behaviour	**Treatment philosophy**	Medical approach emphasizing illness and cure
Individual takes active responsibility for understanding and changing their own behaviour	**Role of client**	Individual is dependent on external forces in the habit-change process
Choice of goal: abstinence or controlled use	**Treatment goal**	Abstinence is the only goal
Cognitive behaviour therapy with the emphasis on the process of change and of the possible achievement of self-control	**Treatment approach**	Confronting the individual into accepting their addiction is based on physiological processes beyond their control and offers group support to reinforce this

of different approaches. However its assumptions about addictive patterns based on empirical findings have given a practical framework for working towards more realistic goals.

The central assumption of RP is that substance abuse is a learned, maladaptive behaviour pattern which, for the individual, becomes the main way of coping. RP implies that the person is capable of change and self-control and that alternative coping strategies are needed to achieve either abstinence or controlled use. This model requires that treatment has an educational approach whereby therapists enable individuals to identify their own particular 'high risk situations' (situations that lead to heavy or uncontrolled use). Also, it promotes the learning and practising of skills necessary to prevent relapse and maintain lifestyle changes. It also favours the self-management approach whereby the client is the agent of change and can therefore learn and implement alternative coping skills.

RP makes the important distinction between lapse (some substance use after an attempt to abstain or reduce consumption) and relapse (the return to previous uncontrolled use pattern) addressing the attributions made when the treatment goal is violated (goal violation effect) and how the client's cognitions can be challenged to prevent a lapse from becoming a relapse. The psychological theory and research findings providing the foundations of this model are given in the essential text by Marlatt & Gordon (1985). Table 7.2 gives a summary of the goals of RP.

RP and management, as intervention strategies are targeted at individuals in the action, maintenance and relapse stages as illustrated. These provide the most useful interventions for facilitating long-term change.

High risk situations

The original analysis of lapse situations by Marlatt and colleagues (Cummings, Gordon and Marlatt, 1980) was based on the experiences of different groups; 'alcoholics', smokers, heroin 'addicts' as well as 'compulsive gamblers' and 'dieters', and identified two broad categories of high risk situations:

- intrapersonal – situations relating to internal states;
- interpersonal – situations relating to interaction with others.

Table 7.3 describes the categories in more detail.

Table 7.2 Goals of relapse prevention

- To increase personal confidence and choice
- To enable clients to anticipate, avoid or/and manage high risk situations
- To teach clients behavioural and cognitive coping skills to manage high risk situations and lapses
- To increase understanding about personal patterns of thought, feelings and behaviour that may lead to lapse or relapse
- To teach clients with strategies to prevent a lapse from becoming a full-blown relapse
- To promote a positive lifestyle change focusing on achieving balance between stressful and pleasurable activities

---

Table 7.3 High risk situations

Intrapersonal	Interpersonal
1 Negative emotional states	6 Interpersonal conflicts
2 Negative physical states	7 Social pressure
3 Positive emotional states	8 Positive emotion states
4 Testing personal control	
5 Urges and temptations	

Negative emotional states, interpersonal conflict and social pressure, account for most lapses. It is important to acknowledge that high risk situations are often complex events that may involve intrapersonal as well as interpersonal factors. There is often a sequence or chain of events that leads to a high risk situation, where the individual may make a series of decisions over a period of time, seemingly irrelevant decisions that can lead to a lapse.

In one of the RP groups, for example, a woman described a situation were she had found herself at an off licence buying a bottle of wine and she could not understand how she got there. She was asked in detail about the events on that day, how she had felt and what she had done, and she was able to identify that she had woken up craving for alcohol and that she proceeded to have a very stressful day. She had decided to take a different route home because she wanted to buy cigarettes. She had gone into the off-licence seemingly wanting to buy cigarettes, despite the fact that she had a full packet in her pocket. By establishing the high risk factors and the seemingly irrelevant decisions she had taken she was able to understand the events that led her to buying the bottle of wine. This sequence of events is referred to as a 'set-up' and clients are encouraged to trace their steps to tease out the decisions and events that lead to the lapse. This process of self-awareness is the first step to being able to discuss alternative coping plans. If a lapse has occurred, cognitive strategies enable the client to reframe attributions for lapse from guilt and self-blame (e.g. 'I am a failure; I cannot stop') to being retributed to external and controllable factors (e.g. 'It was a difficult situation to handle') thus the lapse is seen as a mistake in the learning process. From identifying the high risk factors the client is able to discuss strategies for preparing for risk and building confidence for a new lifestyle. The above forms the basis for RP and the next section of this chapter will focus on how these can be implemented on an outpatient programme.

Individual counselling

RP is a useful model for individual counselling, as an adjunct to group work, as well as in addressing the long-term maintenance strategies. Identifying and planning for high risk situations, as well as focusing on the individual lifestyle changes, is essential work with individuals in the 'maintenance stage'. The use of questionnaires such as 'the inventory of drinking situations and the situational confidence questionnaire' (Annis, 1982a, 1982b) are useful tools to compile individual profiles of high risk situations and of self-efficacy ratings over these situations. These questionnaires are used in the groups, but clients are encouraged to discuss them in more detail with their keyworker. Cognitive behavioural strategies such as described in the counselling guide by Trower, Casey and Dryden (1988) are essential to address such areas as cognitive distortions.

Group programme

Setting up the group

As part of a community alcohol team, groups are organized to participate in rolling programmes lasting seven weeks. Two members of staff with experience in running the group meet to notify staff and clients of the starting date, arrange assessment interviews, and gather and organize group material based on established topics. A new member of the team who wants to learn the model may also join as the third therapist and takes an equal part in the preparation and the group delivery. The group is organized to last for two and a half hours once a week for seven weeks.

Structure of the group

A detailed account of the structure and techniques is found in Wanigaratne, *et al.* (1990). This structure has been developed further to include a space to work on individual goals and group interaction. It is important to use this framework to respond to the client material without worrying too much about adhering to a rigid structure. There is also the added flexibility that has meant that certain topics that are more relevant to a particular group can be given more attention.

A handout (Table 7.4) is given to clients at the assessment interview. It previews the topics to be covered at the group programme. In the first hour the group concentrates on reviewing personal goals discussed at the first meeting. These goals may relate to drinking or may relate to other aspects of a person's life. These goals are broken down into weekly steps which are rated and reviewed every week. Each member of the group has equal time and the group members are encouraged to make suggestions and discuss strategies for achieving the goals. This is an opportunity for members of the group to get to know each other, to give each other feedback and for therapists to highlight coping strategies and individual resources with the aim of raising self-efficacy. The second half of the group session is spent on introducing a topic, with discussion on personal experiences and views, and usually involves either a written exercise or role play. Coping skills are discussed and handouts summarizing a particular topic and a recommended task to take home. Useful cognitive behavioural material for working with problem drinkers is described by Monti *et al.*, (1989) which can be easily introduced into the group programme.

Table 7.4 Information sheet on the relapse prevention group

The relapse prevention group is a short course of seven two-hour sessions, with a break for refreshments. The aim of this course is to focus on changes, in the way you think, the way you cope with feelings and the changes in behaviour, necessary for you to change your drinking pattern.

The group will be held at : (address)

Dates: Tuesday from 10.00 am to 12.30 pm

1. 1st March Introduction: goal setting: overview of the course: urges and cravings
2. 8th March Lapse, relapse and rule violation
3. 15th March High risk situations and set-ups
4. 22nd March Dealing with difficult emotions, depression, anger
5. 29th March Anxiety management
6 5th April Lifestyle balance
7. 12th April Decision-making – summary of the course and where to go from here.

Please arrive at 9.45 am for 10.00 am start

We look forward to seeing you. If you have any queries please contact (Course leaders) on (telephone number)
We recommend that you attend all group sessions to get the best from the course. The only expectation we have is for you to attend alcohol free on the day (and the previous evening) of the group, regardless of your current goal

The principles are from other therapeutic models that have been incorporated to enhance RP. The problem-solving approach has offered certain techniques for addressing goal setting that go beyond the drinking behaviour and are useful when trying to help clients make gradual changes in their lifestyle. Group psychotherapy theories (Yalom, 1985) have given a framework for paying attention to 'dynamic' interactions which occur in groups. Discussing some of these interactions in supervision assists therapists to explore difficulties in trying to facilitate the group.

Selection criteria and assessment process

The optimum number of clients per group is six to eight. It has been found that to achieve this number around 15 clients need to be interviewed in order to be left with a core of eight. Attrition can be due to many factors but this usually occurs because clients may have changed their minds about the group or may have other commitments which clash (i.e. work, holidays, hospital appointments). Some clients may have resumed drinking and may require other interventions such as detoxification subsequent to starting the group. Outpatient work requires flexibility and constant review of plans as client circumstances are often changing.

Clients who are felt to be most appropriate for the group are those individuals that have experienced relapses in the past or those that are finding it difficult to change their lifestyle. Although RP can be carried out individually, the group experience usually adds the opportunity of mutual learning which is in itself an empowering experience for most clients. Those who are unsure about their drinking goal may also join the group with the aim of clarifying whether they need to control drink or abstain. But most importantly we offer the programme to all clients and the basic criteria is that the clients want to attend. One of the most important factors in the successful recruitment of clients is that all team members actively promote awareness and usefulness of the group as an addition to individual work.

Exclusions

The only clients that do not benefit from the group programme are those who have literacy problems or those with a disability that may make it difficult for them to benefit from the group, such as severe visual or auditory impairment. Severe memory impairment or an inability to concentrate and sit for an hour may also exclude some clients, but usually clients experiencing such difficulties require residential treatment. However the structure of the group has been found to be helpful for some clients with memory deficits.

Assessment interview

The assessment for the group is arranged, optimally within two weeks of the date set for the group to start. This usually lasts for approximately half an hour and has a structured interview format. Both therapists arrange to meet with each client with the following aims:

- to establish rapport and reduce dropout from the group;
- for clients to have an opportunity to clarify expectations and to discuss any anxieties about joining a group;
- to discuss current drinking goals (i.e. abstinence, controlled drinking or not sure) and to rate their current confidence in achieving that goal;
- to discuss any other concerns, treatment plans and what they would like to get from attending the group.

This is also an opportunity to discuss practicalities e.g. getting to the group on time, the need for additional support such as supervised disulfiram, sick notes and letters to employers. If clients feel they are not able to commit to the seven weeks they are offered to attend the next group programme. This interview can also be used to review the intensity of the treatment needed. For example, it may be that the client may require an intensive structured day or residential programme, and the therapist may use this opportunity to help the client decide on the best treatment option.

This structured interview format has been shown to reduce the dropout rate for attendance at a relapse prevention group (Keaney *et al.*, 1995). It is important to point out that most clients wanting help feel very anxious and hesitant about joining a group and will often do so after they have established a trusting relationship with their key-worker. Their informed advice and encouragement is crucial. Clients find it easier to join the RP group because it is referred to as a 'course' which offers learning rather than something more threatening.

Follow-up group

The follow-up group, is held once a month for one and a half hour and this is an open group for all the clients that have attended the group programmes. Clients are sent a letter once a month giving a reminder of the day and time. This provides a forum for clients to discuss lifestyle changes, high risk situations as well as lapses and relapses. Some clients choose to attend monthly and others less frequently, and some attend in crisis requesting additional treatment. The format of the group is simple and it involves all the clients having a space to discuss changes. The therapist offers support and reinforcement of the model. This is the point at which RP is really put to work and where clients begin to sustain longitudinal perspective of the change process. Also this low intensity group commitment allows individuals to have an opportunity to keep up vigilance, and most importantly to continue giving each other support and encouragement through difficulties.

At one of the follow-up groups, several clients discussed difficulties and some had lapsed. One client explained that he had been abstinent for a year but had attended a funeral at which he had had several drinks. Although he felt disappointed he said that he was able to stop and not allow that day to develop into a drinking binge, and other group members praised him for his ability to prevent a relapse. Another client discussed an overwhelming urge for alcohol after 15 months of abstinence and said that he had rung the keyworker from the pub to prevent a lapse. At the end of the group, a new client said that she had felt very depressed about her recent relapse and that she had not wanted to attend the group. She felt she had let people down but said 'I am pleased I came because I realise that it's not easy for anyone and that you all find it as difficult, and I feel more positive about carrying on'. For clients who have a long history of dependence on alcohol, there may be a need for ongoing support in their first two years of abstinence which could support them either individually or in a group situation.

Benefits and limitations of RP group programmes

The group experience offers an opportunity for sharing common experiences of problem behaviour patterns and to exchange ideas on how these can be changed. Usually clients feel misunderstood and isolated in their experience and it is of immense support to have an opportunity to feel that they are not 'the only ones' and to have a sense of belonging. The benefits of group therapy have long been recognized, and it is important to acknowledge the psychotherapeutic benefits of group therapy. To facilitate groups requires an understanding of group processes and group psychotherapy principles and benefits, such as those outlined by Yalom (1985), that can enhance the cognitive behavioural work.

The emphasis of RP is on the process of changing lifestyles, which requires certain skills and strategies, but the impact on personal identity is often discussed as well by group members. The clients experience a major upheaval when they decide to change their drinking pattern, which affects them at different levels; emotional, cognitive, behavioural and physiological. Clients are able to discuss the effort that is required to change the 'old way' of being and how, sometimes, it is easier to revert back to their familiar lifestyles, even if this is destructive. By acknowledging this 'struggle' in behaviour change clients are able to accept more realistic expectations and not to be devastated if they lapse. The group is able to offer individuals more information and opportunities for learning from other clients which is a major advantage over individual counselling. RP allows them to address the similarities but also recognize the individual constellation of risk factors and resources. There is great advantage in individuals having different goals (controlled drinking, reduction or abstinence) which places an emphasis on personal choice and allows clients to come to their own conclusions. Most clients feel ambivalent about their goals, and the fact that they have a choice usually precipitates their individual decision.

As the focus is on cognitions and behaviours, clients and therapists are able to give constructive feedback without criticism of the individual. Shared concepts, such as set-ups and cognitive distortions, are highlighted with the aim of increasing awareness. However, as RP is a structured programme, it offers a safe environment of low emotional intensity. It is possible to discuss difficult and painful experiences as trust is developed over the seven weeks. This means that this is an excellent introduction to group therapy that is non-threatening, and clients are able to then make informed choices about other treatment options.

Over the seven weeks and as the different topics are covered, assessment of individual risks areas and particular difficulties is made. This often points to areas in which the client may benefit from additional treatment and this is fed back at the end of the group and suggestions are made on the most appropriate next step.

Difficulties with RP groups

One of the main difficulties about the group programme is that it is never long enough to cover all the material. Initially when starting to work with this model one feels the urgency to cover everything and this often leads to bombarding the clients with too much information. Over time, it has been found that it is important to pay attention to key concepts which are often repeated. Table 7.5 describes the essential features of RP which is what we aim to cover by the end of each group.

Another difficulty with group work is that trusting relationships do develop as the programme progresses and great sadness is expressed when the group programme is coming to an end. Therapists often feel tempted to extend the group,

Table 7.5 Key features of relapse prevention

1 Assessment of risk	Analysis of personal high risk situations
2 Planning for risk	Ways of avoiding or coping with potential high risk situations
3 Responding to risk	Goal violation effect difference between lapse and relapse
4 Lifestyle balance	
5 Promoting the model	Awareness of self-management and vigilance

but there is an acknowledgement that group members may need to address different issues in the longer term. This is why we have ongoing groups targeted to specific goals which clients are encouraged to attend i.e. weekly abstinence support or controlled drinking group. Stress and anxiety management is an area that is often identified and a separate stress management course has been developed to enhance the RP group programme.

In RP therapists need to be skilled in group work and to be able to promote understanding and learning at different levels. Some clients may want to discuss ideas in great depth and others may find this difficult. The skill is in paying enough attention to individual needs as well as eliciting the common themes.

CONCLUSION

Nurses working in the community have a responsibility for keyworking and case management. Individual counselling, group work and RP can offer a framework for all of these functions. As the emphasis of this model is on awareness and learning, it is necessary for nurses to have an educational and facilitative role. They 'teach' certain concepts but these can only be made relevant and useful through interaction with the clients' experience. The clients' own resources are valued and encouraged: thus, nurses and clients are working in partnership. The theoretical material offered to clients is meaningless unless they are actively involved in the change process. Therefore, nurses do not expect clients to assume a passive or 'patient role' but are viewed as being capable and responsible for their changes.

In the case management of clients, lapses and relapses are framed as learning episodes even though we cannot ignore that these are still distressing events. Nurses are required to assume a problem-solving function and access clients to the appropriate treatment. For example, in relapse crisis clients are offered quick access to outpatient detoxification with the aim of minimizing the harm of relapse. Clients are encouraged to make contact with the service, and successful outpatient care is regarded as positive relapse management. Thus, the fact that clients can reduce the length of their relapse can be viewed as a step forward.

REFERENCES

Allsop, S. and Saunders, W. (1989) Relapse and alcohol problems, in *Relapse and Addictive Behaviour* (ed. M. Gossop), Tavistock/Routledge, London.

Annis, H.M. (1982a) *Inventory of Drinking Situations*, Addiction Research Foundation, Ontario, Canada.

Annis, H.M. (1982b) *Situational Confidence Questionnaire*, Addiction Research Foundation, Ontario, Canada.

Annis, H.M. and Davis, C.S. (1987) Self-efficacy and the prevention of alcoholic relapse: initial findings from a treatment trial, in *Addictive disorders: Psychological research on assessment and treatment* (eds T.B. Baker and T. Cannon), Praeger, New York.

Annis, H.M. and Peachey, J.E. (1992) The use of calcium carbamide in relapse prevention counselling: results of a randomized controlled trial. *British Journal Of Addiction*, **87**(1), 63–72.

Bandura, A. (1977) Self-efficacy: Toward a unifying theory of behaviour change. *Psychological Review*, **84**(2), 191–215.

Cummings, C., Gordon, J.R. and Marlatt, G.A. (1980) Relapse: strategies of prevention and prediction, in *The Addictive Behaviours: treatment of alcoholism, drug abuse, smoking and obesity* (ed. W.R. Miller), Pergamon Press, Oxford, pp. 291–321.

Gorski, T.T. (1986) Relapse Prevention Training: A new recovery tool. *Alcohol Health and Research World*, **11**(1), 6–11.

Gorski, T.T. (1990) The cenaps model of relapse prevention: Basic principles and procedures. *Journal of Psychoactive Drugs*, **22**(2), 125–33.

Hodgson, R.J. and Rankin, H.J. (1982) Cue exposure and relapse prevention, in *Clinical case studies in the behavioural treatment of alcoholism* (eds W.M. Hay and P.E. Nathan), Plenum Press, New York, pp. 207–48.

Keaney, F., Wanigaratne, S. and Pullin, J. (1995) The use of structured assessment interview as an intervention to reduce drop-out rates in the out patient relapse prevention groups for problem drinkers. *The International Journal of Addiction*, **30**(10), 1355–62.

Lindstrom, L. (1992) *Alcoholism: matching client to treatment*, Oxford University Press, Oxford.

Marlatt, G.A. (1979) A cognitive-behavioural model of the relapse process. *NIDA Research Monograph*, 25, 191–200.

Marlatt, G.A. and Gordon, J.R. (eds) (1985) Relapse prevention: maintenance strategies in the treatment of addictive behaviours, Guilford Press, New York.

Miller, W.R. (1983) Motivational interviewing with problem drinkers. *Behavioural Psychotherapy*, **11**(2), 147–72.

Miller, W.R. (1985) Motivation for treatment: a review with special emphasis on alcoholism. *Psychological Bulletin*, **98**(1), 84–107.

Miller, W.R. (1989) Matching individuals with interventions, in *Handbook of Alcoholism: Treatment Approaches: Effective alternatives* (eds R.K. Hester and W.R. Miller), Pergamon, New York.

Monti, M., Abrams, D.B., Kadden, R.M. and Cooney, N.L. (1989) *Treating Alcohol Dependence: A coping skills training guide*, Guilford Press, New York.

Prochaska, J.O. and Diclemente, C.C. (1982) Transtheoretical therapy: Toward a more integrative model of change. *Psychotherapy: Theory, research and practice*, **19**, 276–88.

Prochaska, J.O., Diclemente, C.C. and Nocross, J.C. (1992) In search of how people change: Applications to addictive behaviours. *American Psychologist*, **4**(9), 1102–14.

Trower, P., Casey, A. and Dryden, W. (1988) *Cognitive-Behavioural Counselling in Action*, Sage Publications, London.

Wanigaratne, S., Wallace, W., Pullin, J., Keaney, F. and Farmer, R. (1990) *Relapse prevention for addictive behaviours: A manual for therapists*, Blackwell Scientific Publications, Oxford.

Yalom, I.D. (1985) *Theory and Practice of Group Psychotherapy, 3rd edn*, Harper Collins, USA.

8

Psychotherapeutic approaches and nursing interventions

Gary Winship and Clare Unwin

INTRODUCTION

The psychopathology of substance misuse may be defined in terms of a hierarchy of causes ranging from social factors, such as poverty, fashion and peer pressure, to indepth developmental conflicts that lie at the root of substance misuse (Wurmser, 1974). For example, the often used term frozen adolescence connotes a developmental conflict considered to be an indepth factor in continued substance misuse. The association between adolescence and substance misuse is reflected in the nomenclature where substances are described in terms of a surge of excitation, for instance; 'crack', 'smack', 'bang' and 'whizz' to name a few. The notion that misuse arises from a frozen adolescence suggests that some drug users get stuck or fixated with adolescent conflicts, where development becomes frozen and appropriate emotional maturation is prevented. Sexual identity crises, parental/authoritarian problems are just some of the manifestations of a developmental conflict where substance misuse is an attempt to escape or overcome the problems of adolescent conflict.

However, describing substance misuse in terms of an adolescent escapism, does serve to rather trivialize what is otherwise a dangerous and potentially life-threatening pursuit of pleasure. The euphoria of intoxication appears to have a concomitant in the sense of excitement and danger that accompanies using. Substance misusers are aware of the risks associated with drugs; overdosing, accidents and physical illness, as well as psychological damage to self-esteem and personal relationships. It could be argued that danger and death are not incidental in the use of drugs, rather they appear to be intrinsic to the experience. Dependence on psychoactive drugs therefore might be understood psychoanalytically in terms of a death drive acting as the principle motivating force (Bollas, 1991; Holden, 1992). This repetitious enactment of self destructiveness is often part of a lifestyle that courts physical and mental brinkmanship (Joseph, 1982). In examining the aetiology of substance misuse, it is necessary to consider why the user developed such an appetite in the first place.

The aim of this chapter therein, is to explore how depression and destructiveness are manifested in the treatment milieu and how therapeutic encounters may limit self-damage and help the client on the path to recovery. The main theoretical framework explored here is psychodynamic theory and more specifically psychoanalytic and object relations theory. The relevance of object relations theory to nursing is discussed in Fabricius (1993), Attwood (1994) and Winship *et al.*, (1995). The notion of object relations refers to the inner world which might be compared to the set of a 'theatre'. This inner world of people and objects acts upon relations in the external world, at times appearing to offer an internal caveat or life script that influences how events and affairs unfold in current relationships. Object relations offers a model of the fluid interchange between interpersonal and intrapersonal dynamics.

PSYCHOANALYTICAL THEORIES OF ADDICTION

When considering the nature of substance misuse it would appear that there is a dual disposition, that is to say, pleasure and self-destructiveness tend to run a psychical and physical parallel. First, the use of a substance appears to be an attempt to nullify all feelings and thoughts through the creation of a chemically induced pleasurable state of mind (love), and at the same time, the misuse of a drug is itself an expression of a self-destructive drive (hate). This dual disposition could be described as ambivalent – the wish for pleasure while knowing about the dangers. Whether the drug is loved or hated, it becomes the means to a type of psychic retreat from reality. This retreat may be compared to a schizoid process of splitting which predominates in a way that is similar to a psychotic state of mind where fantasy is used as a defensive response to reality (Steiner, 1993). In this respect, the work of Connell (1968) is important because he was one of the first addiction specialists to observe extensively the similarities between psychosis and substance misuse (specifically amphetamines). During consultations with patients who had experienced psychotic states, Connell was always keen to explore indepth the addicts' inner world, attempting to see if any meaning could be discerned in their disturbance. It is this indepth interest in a patient's history that is the fount of a psychodynamic approach and it has been argued that all patients have a right to an indepth psychoanalytical exploration of their substance misuse (Cawley, 1993; Jackson and Williams, 1994).

The use of a substance as a defensive response to reality, where the effect of the substance creates an idealized experience, led Rosenfeld (1965) to postulate that the drug starts to represent an idealized object in the addict's mind. The drug and its effect, by creating a heightened hallucinatory state, become split from reality and act as a defence against anxiety or persecutory feelings. This intoxicated state reinforces the mechanisms of splitting and denial of depression (Fairbairn, 1940;

Grotstein and Rinsley, 1994). Rosenfeld surmized that the existence of these type of schizoid splitting mechanisms in his patients indicated that the developmental root cause of addiction lay at the point when these mechanisms first emerged. Klein (1940, 1946) postulated that splitting and denial emerge during the first few months of life when the infant attempts to expel bad experiences or sensations (feeling cold, hungry, afraid etc.) in order to recapitulate good experiences of pleasure (feeding, nurturing, motherly warmth etc.). Following Klein, Rosenfeld (1965) saw drug addiction as a manifestation of unresolved conflicts from these primary stages of development. This indepth conceptualization of substance misuse might be well described as a theory of frozen infancy when there is a love hunger which becomes addictively quenched by a substance.

So, is it possible to compare the experience of intoxication with that of the experience in infancy of an ideal feeding state? It is interesting to note that many drug users describe the feeling of using as instant gratification. Intoxication with many substances serves to suppress appetite and most drug users tend to be underweight, with the exception of some problem drinkers. It is almost a ubiquitous phenomenon that withdrawal from some psychoactive substances is concomitant with an increase in an appetite for food and most recovering substance misusers put on weight during treatment. One deduction is that the heightened experience of using a drug defends against an experience of depression linked to a primitive hunger for the feeling of being loved and fated. Disturbances in formative experiences, perhaps where anxiety has been ineffectively tolerated, or where there has been poor parental empathy in recognizing infantile needs – may be some of the root causes of a state of frozen infancy. This is a similar line of argument to that of Kohut (1971), where he describes that a defective empathy on the part of the parent/mother may be a root cause of disturbances. These may later surface in problems with substances that act as a replacement for the unfulfilled love from childhood. Some of these psychodynamics are highlighted in the following case vignette.

Case vignette

During the course of 30 weeks of residential treatment C's history unfolded (age 26 years). She said she had been born out of wedlock and, as a result, her mother had made her wear a crucifix upside down and told her she was the devil's daughter. Among C's early memories she recalled being beaten and locked in a cupboard, a punishment that she described as growing to like; 'the safety of the dark cupboard'. She also recalled being teased with food from as early as the age of four. Her mother would put a plateful of food in front of her and then take it away when she would go to eat it. She had difficulties at school and did not learn to read or write. At 14 years of age she became pregnant and soon after giving birth her daughter was taken into permanent care. Her adolescence and young adulthood was characterized by a chaotic pattern of polydrug misuse, followed by a series of violent relationships with men and serious suicide attempts. During the early weeks of her admission to a residential recovery centre it was noted also that she had a disordered pattern of eating which featured binging and vomiting. As a result she was grossly underweight. She would often joke about this and say that she should be called 'little Miss Bones'.

Her physical wellbeing, in terms of her drug use, was stabilized within a few days of admission and her use of injectable drugs was replaced by a steady reducing dose of oral methadone. She remained severely depressed and made threats of self harm of increasing seriousness. A crisis meeting was called by her fellow residents and some members argued that she should be transferred to a psychiatric unit for her own safety. Others felt that she should be allowed to stay but with certain provisos. There was a lengthy discussion following which there was a vote (the unit was organized along the democratic lines akin to a therapeutic community (Crozier, 1979). The vote was split but the majority decided in favour of her staying. Her stay was on the understanding that C would adhere to the community norms and rules (no self harm).

In the following weeks the group vigorously confronted C about, among other things, her eating; 'if you don't eat you'll waste away' she was told. It was the first time that she had been confronted openly in the group about her eating. The staff were sure that she would be unable to bear the confrontation and that she would leave. However she stayed. One of the staff said it was as if she had 'swallowed some of the group's love'. Her progress over the following month was steady as she began to engage with the community taking on more senior roles and responsibilities.

In the kitchen one evening she was preparing a communal dinner. I spoke to her about her plans for an eventual move to a drug rehabilitation unit in the west country and about forming new relationships. She said that she could 'never trust anyone again after that woman' (she always referred to her mother as 'that woman'). She was angry and dismissive of my attempt at suggesting there may be some good opportunities in the future. I pointed this out to her. She replied; 'When something's good I can't cope with it and I have to make it bad'. It seemed that C's good internal objects, fragile though they were, somehow had to be continually poisoned and attacked, even the idea of something possibly being good in the future had to be poisoned. It was as if she could not allow herself to experience anything good and nurturing, and it seemed as if her mother was still torturing her with food. In the kitchen that evening, I felt a familiar feeling of my words being ignored, as if she could not distinguish between something nurturing and something bad.

During her last three weeks of the treatment programme she became more energetic around the unit as she took on senior roles becoming ward representative for the first time. In her last group there was a new patient with a severe eating disorder who was struggling to stay in treatment. When this patient said that she could not bear to stay any longer and that she was going to leave C turned to her and said; 'Y'know you've got to swallow your pride and take in the good with the bad'. It was as if C was articulating that she had found the belief, from somewhere, that something good could exist inside and be held onto. Three years later C came back to the unit's annual party for ex-residents having been drug free ever since. She had completed an extended programme at a rehabilitation unit and was using the extended support of NA in the community. She was as stable as she could remember.

Vignette discussion

The occasion when the group was split over whether C should stay or go was a pivotal moment. On the one hand, the group appeared inclined to eject and punish her and, on the other hand, inclined to meet her need for a good containing mother. This group dynamic, reflected something of C's persecutory internal object relations – notably the haunting spectre of her damaging mother. According to Yalom (1975), the group recapitulated C's source of family conflict. The group unknowingly became torn between acting like C's hostile and rejecting mother and a good new mother concerned about her wellbeing. The ambivalence that C felt inside towards anything good, was mirrored in the ambivalent split enacted in the group as some of the members wanted to expel her while others wanted to contain her. In group dynamic terms this situation was an example of object relations expressed in a group.

For C, her continued drug use meant that whatever residue of a good internal sense of self that she might have had, became increasingly dominated by self-destructive drives. The substances she had used were an attempt to fill a relationship hunger that had been unsatisfied early in her childhood. The frustration and pain that she felt in her life was, on the one hand, defended against by the idealized use of numbing psychoactive substances, while at the same time an expression of her self-destructiveness. The process of therapy was one of repairing the damaging cycle of self-destruction into which she was unconsciously locked, and pointing out to C when she was hurting the good new things in her life. The synthesis of a new inner 'good enough' mother, not perfect but adequate to sustain, appeared to take root in the intensive treatment. This offered her the opportunity to rebuild her inner world afresh as she freed herself from her damaging internal images. The process of becoming attached to the community was a new experience of being loved and cared for which offered her the chance of a new beginning. The theoretical frame for this type of process has been explained by Bowlby and Balint (Pedder, 1976). However, beyond theory, the process of recovery for C is perhaps best explained in the poem that she composed (dictated) for the hospital magazine during the final weeks of her treatment.

'Those Skeletons of You: When you have shut the cupboard door/ And then secured the lock/ You think you've shut those bones away/ Believe me you have not//. If you think they'll stay hidden/ Then you're in for a shock/ As no cupboard door can keep them in/ Even with a lock//. You'll never, ever, hide them/ No matter how you try/ They'll always cause you sorrow/ Until the day you die//. When you least expect them/ They'll sneak up from behind/ It's a sad but simple fact/ That the past is seldom kind//. So don't hide them in the cupboards/ Or keep them out of sight/ Once they're out they fade away/ Old bones don't like the light.'

Psychosocial-analysis

The source of C's substance misuse lay in her disturbed formative experiences. A psychoanalytic model of development attends closely to the experience of primary dependency and the emergence of interdependency. This is when individuality is not the starting point of life, but that which emerges from an intricate experience of dependency on others (Rustin, 1991). These early experiences lay the foundations for those relationships to follow. This model of development interlaces psychoanalytic theory with social theory and would seem to be apposite to working with substance misusers where the dependency on a drug is shifted to a dependency on others during the process of treatment.

It has often been interesting to note how clients during treatment shift their attachment/dependency from drugs on to their therapist and peers. Balint (1968) has described how the therapeutic relationship has the potential to engender dependency in the patient. A psychoanalytical approach is often criticized for fostering dependency, however, it is more accurate to say that a psychoanalytic approach accepts the reality of a need for dependency that the patient presents. The fear of dependency is often a preponderant force that undermines the efficacy of many treatment approaches. Pedder (1991) has discussed these issues and is critical of the denigration of dependency treatment within psychiatric services. He notes that other cultures have a more reasonable acceptance of dependency and suggests that the west may learn from some these. From a psychotherapeutic perspective, the starting point of recovery is not one of fostering dependency, but rather one of allowing it to emerge as a concomitant of therapy. The transitional process of a shifting of dependency from a drug onto a therapist is illustrated in the following vignette.

Case vignette

M, a heroin addict in his early 30s, underwent quite a difficult withdrawal. The symptoms of withdrawal were exacerbated by severe headaches. Attempts to control the headaches using hot baths, tiger balm, herbal teas were all unsuccessful. While the headaches were a symptom of withdrawal they also appeared to be associated with a craving for heroin (pain relief). As a last resort M was prescribed paracetamol. His use of paracetamol only lasted a couple of days. His headaches soon lessened in intensity. After several weeks he had begun to settle well into the treatment programme. He eventually progressed on to a day pass which meant he was able to leave the unit unaccompanied. However, while out on his first day pass he craved for drugs and came close to using. When he returned to the unit he reported that when he had craved drugs and had been tempted to use, he had been surprised by an image in his mind of his key worker rushing down the ward, carrying two paracetamol in a beaker to give to him. This image, he said, was related to his early experience when he was undergoing detoxification.

Vignette discussion

The image in M's mind was significant insofar as it appeared to represent something of how he had internalized his key worker. It showed the transitional process between relying on, and investing in a drug, and how this was transferred to the key worker. In M's mind, there appeared to be an interrelationship between the objects of the beaker, the drugs and the key worker. M appeared to have internalized his experiences of the caring key worker and this had helped him deal with his feelings of craving. M's task during treatment was to re-evaluate his dependence on substances. In the early part of his admission he believed that the only intervention that would help him was a chemical one. Therefore, he had 'split-off' and denied the real significance of the care and support that he received from the staff and his key worker. His therapy was a process of acknowledging that the real experience of his contact with his key worker was that which had the potential to sustain him, and not the rather insignificant paracetamol relief. In this case, the task of the staff was to help M see how he had 'split-off' the human help that he had received and accredited it to the paracetamol.

CONCLUSION

The vignettes illustrate how pivotal the interpersonal relationship between the therapist and the client became. A psychodynamic approach, when the transference dynamics between the nurse and the patient are considered as the basis for the therapeutic encounter, has been explored by Strang (1982). Strang emphasized that the process of detoxification was not so much about the biological process of withdrawal, but rather about overcoming the client's resistance to treatment by de-medicalizing the process through the institution of a humane interpersonal therapeutic process. He observed that the dual role of nurse within the therapeutic milieu – social contact intermingled with formal individual therapeutic contact – provided a helpful blurring of the role of the nurse therapist. Citing Freud's concept of positive transference, Strang conceived of a ward milieu where the everyday events were the basis for healthy interactions.

Most substance misusers struggle, with varying levels of success, to deal with negative emotional states, i.e. feelings of sadness, loss and separation and these states have been shown to be those which are the most likely cause of a relapse following treatment (Marlatt and Gordon, 1985). The process of therapy therefore involves the experience of being with a negative emotional state without the continuous and nullifying prop of chemical support. Events which involve facing sadness and loss are opportunities for therapeutic encounters as in real life. Disappointment and sadness do not need to be faced when one is fixated on the next hit just around the corner, all disappointment can be focused on a substance. The process of therapy therefore offers a kind of reality confrontation at the same time as offering the reassurance of commonality of experience with peers who are undergoing similar experiences. The therapeutic encounter enables the conflict to be shared collectively, that is to say, with the therapist and with peers. The bad and unwanted aspects of the self may be contained either by the individual therapist or the group (or both in treatment centres that offer a combined treatment approach of group and individual therapy) before being reintegrated in a way that exerts less disturbance.

From a psychoanalytic perspective it is the process of bringing into consciousness, from unconsciousness, painful previous experiences usually associated with family conflicts, which can then be seen and evaluated. The pain cannot be extinguished but it can be processed and thereby diminished. Internally, the object relationships are transformed when a persecutory self object is mitigated by a more benign self-disposition, as in C's case where the persecutory mother was superseded by the construction of a more caring internal mother.

The emphasis on relational and intersubjective experiences between clients and staff suggests that the basis of a nursing approach might embrace the type of interpersonal model of nursing described by Peplau (1952; 1988). Peplau (1994) has recently re-asserted that the future of psychiatric nursing lies in the endeavour of the nurse to develop the capacity to act as the agent of change. Therefore, if we approach addiction from this social perspective, then the fundamental principle of treatment should emphasize an understanding of the importance of the relationship between the substance misuser and others – therapist/counsellor or peers (Kaufman, 1990; Winick, 1991). Broadly speaking, this is the basis of a psychodynamic approach whereby the relationship between the addict and their influencing network of relations, past and present, is explored in depth through the shared experience of the nurse/patient alliance.

REFERENCES

Attwood, A. (1994) What did we talk about last week? – a study of forgetting in one schizophrenic and two borderline clients in counselling. *Psychodynamic Counselling*, **1**(1), 46–64.

Balint, M. (1968) *The Basic Fault*, Tavistock, London.

Bollas, C. (1991) *Forces of Destiny. Psychoanalysis and the Human Idiom*, Free Association Books, London.

Cawley, R.H. (1993) Psychiatry is more than a science. *British Journal of Psychiatry*, **162**, 154–60.

Connell, P.H. (1968) The use and abuse of Amphetamines. *The Practitioner*, **200**(196), 234–43.

Crozier, A. (1979) *Attempts at democracy. In Therapeutic Communities – Reflections and Progress* (eds R.D. Hinshelwood and N. Manning), Routledge, London, pp. 263–71.

Fabricius, J. (1993) *Psychodynamic Perspectives, in Mental Health Nursing* (eds H. Wright and M. Giddey), Chapman and Hall, London, pp. 44–55.

Fairbairn, W.R.D. (1940) *Schizoid Factors in the Personality, in Psychoanalytic Studies of the Personality 1952*, Tavistock, London, pp. 3–27.

Grotstein, J.S. and Rinsley, D.B. (eds) (1994) *Fairbairn and the Origins of Object Relations*, Free Association Books, London.

Holden, R.J. (1992) The death drive exemplified in a case alcohol dependence. *Journal of Clinical Nursing*, **1**(4), 213–17.

Jackson, M. and Williams, P. (1994) *Unimaginable Storms*, Karnac Books, London.

Joseph, B. (1982) Addiction to near death. *International Journal of Psychoanalysis*, **63**(part 4), 449–56.

Kaufman, E. (1990) Critical aspects of the psychodynamics of substance abuse and the evaluation of their application to a psychotherapeutic approach. *The International Journal of Addictions*, **25**(2), 97–116.

Klein, M. (1940) Mourning and it's Relation to Manic-Depressive States, in *Contributions to Psycho-Analysis, 1921–1945* (1948), Hogarth, London.

Klein, M. (1946) Notes on Some Schizoid Mechanisms, in *Envy and Gratitude and Other Works 1946–1963*, (1988) Virago, London, pp. 1–24.

Kohut, H. (1971) *The Analysis of the Self*, University Press, New York.

Marlatt, G.A. and Gordon, J.R. (1985) *Relapse Prevention: Maintenance Strategies In the Treatment of Addictive Behaviour*, Guilford Press, New York.

Pedder, J.R. (1976) Attachment and New Beginning. Some link between the work of Michael Balint and John Bowlby. *International Review of Psycho-Analysis*, **3**, 491–7.

Pedder, J.R. (1991) Fear of dependency in therapeutic relationships. *British Journal of Medical Psychology*, **64**(part 2), 117–26.

Peplau, H (1952) *Interpersonal Relations in Nursing*, Putnam, New York.

Peplau, H (1988) *Selected Works. Interpersonal Theory in Nursing*, Singer, New York.

Peplau, H (1994) Psychiatric mental health nursing. *Journal of Psychiatric and Mental Health Nursing*, **1**(1), 3–7.

Rosenfeld, H. (1965) *Psychotic States*, Hogarth Press, London.

Rustin, M. (1991) *The Good Society and the Inner World*, Verso, London.

Steiner, R. (1994) 'The Tower of Babel' or After Babel in Contemporary Psychoanalysis? *International Journal of Psychoanalysis*, (December) 75 (Parts 5–6), 883–901.

Strang, J. (1982) Psychotherapy by nurses – some special characteristics. *Journal of Advanced Nursing*, **7**, 167–71.

Winick, C. (1991) The counsellor in drug user treatment. *The International Journal of Addictions*, 25(12) 1479–1502.

Winship, G., Harman, B., Burring, S. *et al.* (1995) Utilising countertransference in the process of nursing drug dependant patients. *Psychoanalytic Psychotherapy*, **9**(2) 195–207.

Wurmser, L. (1974) Psychoanalytic considerations of the etiology of compulsive drug use. *Journal of American Psychoanalytic Association*, **22**(4), 820–43.

Yalom, I.D. (1975) *The Theory and Practice of Group Psychotherapy*, Basic Books, New York.

Complementary therapies in addiction nursing practice

9

Linda McDonald and G. Hussein Rassool

INTRODUCTION

Complementary therapies are gaining increased recognition within the allopathic heathcare system in the UK, and there is a significant interest in the development of its use in nursing specialties. Increasingly, healthcare consumers are looking for non-pharmacological alternatives to conventional healthcare (Thomas *et al.*, 1991; Consumers' Association, 1995). It has been suggested that it is those who are disenchanted with modern medicine rather than the disenfranchized who have turned to complementary medicine (Trevelyan, 1993).

There is a wide range of alternative and complementary therapies being used within the healthcare system. During the last five years, nurses in addiction nursing have shown a growing interest in introducing complementary therapies as part of the treatment regimens: acupuncture, aromatherapy, reflexology and shiatsu are being used as part of interventions strategies or as the primary treatment.

The aims of this chapter are to provide a brief overview of the therapies more likely to be used in the substance misuse field, and there is a selected literature review on the clinical application of these therapies. The focus of the chapter will be based on three complementary therapies: acupuncture, aromatherapy and reflexology. There are other complementary therapies and alternative medicines that are appropriate in clinical practice and for a comprehensive review the reader is referred to the following texts: Vickers (1993); Rankin-Box (1987); Trevelyan and Booth (1994).

HOLISTIC NURSING AND CLINICAL PRACTICE

Complementary therapies are based on the idea of 'holism' in which the client is viewed in terms of the interdependence of his/her medical, psychological, social and spiritual functioning and that none of which takes precedence or dominance over the other. The term 'holistic' is often used interchangeably with complementary therapies.

In complementary therapies healthcare interventions are used according to the clients' needs, unlike the traditional health approaches based on the western scientific paradigm. Engebretson (1992) stated that the holistic health movement is characterized by efforts from healthcare providers and others such as nurses to expand the biomedical model so that alternative modalities of treatment are incorporated. Furthermore, Pfeil (1994) indicated that the emphasis of holism is upon the client and practitioner sharing decision-making and goal-setting so that it is acceptable to both, rather than taking dogmatic approaches to treatment. This paradigm shift from a medical-oriented model to a bio-psychosocial model is reflected in the growing use of complementary therapies. Complementary therapies are a valuable option open to addiction nurses, and it is the right of consumers to make healthcare choices as part of their healthcare options.

Nurses have already successfully incorporated complementary therapies into general nursing practices (Malkin, 1994; Burke and Sikora, 1992; Stevensen, 1992). A survey investigating nurses'(N = 393) views on complementary therapies found that the most popular therapies among nurses were aromatherapy, massage, reflexology and shiatsu (Trevelyan, 1996). Complementary therapies are mainly used by addiction nurses for the purposes of detoxification, massage, relaxation, stress reduction, pain relief and palliative care.

Professional accountability and responsibility

The UKCC (1992) paper on the *Standards for the Administration of Medicines* recognized the growing use of therapies within nursing practice and referred explicitly to the administration of herbal, homeopathic and alternative therapies. Under the title 'Complementary and Alternative Therapies' (para. 39), the paper states that – 'Some registered nurses, midwives and health visitors, having first undertaken successfully a training in complementary therapy which involves the use of substances such as essential oils, apply their specialist knowledge and skill in their practice. It is essential that practice in these respects, as in all others, is based on sound principles, available knowledge and skills. So, too, must the practitioners' personal accountability for his or her professional practice'. Despite guidance from the UKCC (1992), 'nurses need to ensure that their position regarding these therapies is based upon a judicious review of the literature and carefully crafted and reasoned actions' (Gates, 1994).

It is clear from these statements that education and training must be undertaken by nurses in order to use complementary therapies within their professional practice. Rankin-Box (1991) suggested that those therapists claiming to treat or cure certain ailments on the basis of anecdotal evidence as opposed to definitive research evidence may leave themselves open to ethical, legal and professional concern.

In terms of procedure and the incorporation of complementary therapies within healthcare interventions, it is essential that clinical practice is based on professional competencies. The importance of consent to the use of such treatments must also be recognized. Stevensen (1992) suggested having a formal consent form for clients to sign, a printed information sheet for clients and their relatives, and keeping formal records of all clients' comments and reactions to the treatment, as this may form the basis of future research. In the clinical application of complementary therapies, a professional indemnity insurance should be a prerequisite. Most complementary therapies have leading bodies that can offer advice on insurance, education and training.

Acupuncture

Acupuncture, an ancient system of healing , was first described in 'the yellow emperors classic of internal medicine' over 400 years ago and is based on the Chinese philosophy that the body has a network of energy pathways, called 'meridians'. These meridians connect the external surface of the body to the internal allowing the passage of chi. Chi is regarded as the vital energy of all beings, and the fundamental energy of the universe. In human beings, it is the energy that sustains life. If the meridians become blocked the chi will be unable to flow freely causing discord and possible damage to the body. Both physical and psychological problems can cause blockage in the pathways.

The use of auricular acupuncture in the treatment of substance misuse was pioneered in The Lincoln Hospital in New York in the early 1970s . It is used to treat most forms of substance misuse and addictive behaviours; cigarette smoking (Low, 1977; Chen, 1979), alcoholism (Smith, 1979), methadone detoxification (Gomez and Mikhail, 1974), detoxification of opiate, cocaine, crack cocaine, alcohol and tobacco addiction (Smith and Khan, 1988), and preventing relapse (Katims *et al.*, 1992).

There is evidence to suggest that the efficacy of acupuncture as a substance misuse treatment with problem drinkers is limited. For instance, a study by Worner *et al.*, (1992) concluded that with a small racially mixed sample of alcoholics, standard acupuncture did not improve outcome in terms of AA attendance, completion of treatment and number of relapses. The reason for the paucity of acupuncture detoxification therapy is not merely a lack of understanding of its physiologic basis of action, but primarily the scarcity of controlled objective clinical studies and failure to describe acupuncture in quantitative objective Western terminology (Katims *et al.*,1992). Auricular acupuncture is not a magic solution to substance misuse treatment, but can be a valuable aid in the detoxification process. The next section will present a case vignette to illustrate the use of auricular acupuncture in a substance misuse agency.

Case vignette – auricular acupuncture

David was referred to a substance misuse agency by his mother who was concerned about his increasing cocaine habit. He was invited to attend the service for assessment. David attended the service on time but was very agitated, restless and with marked pressure of speech. It was increasingly difficult to carry out the assessment and the possibility of using complementary therapy was discussed. David was initially very sceptical, but agreed to treatment. Once the contra-indications of acupuncture were established, the procedure was explained and written consent obtained.

Auricular acupuncture was initiated according to the agency's policy on the use of complementary therapies. Within 10 minutes, David displayed no signs of agitation enabling the assessment to proceed. David continued to attend the agency on a daily basis for acupuncture, support and counselling. This illustrates the benefits of auricular acupuncture, at the pre-assessment stage but not as a primary treatment.

Aromatherapy

The benefits of aromatic plants have been known to man for centuries. Around 3 500 BC, the priestesses of ancient Egypt used the burning of resin and gum of certain plants to clear the mind. In Roman times essential oils were used in massage. By the 20th century, aromatherapy was introduced in the UK and Europe in a range of healthcare settings. In 1937 a French chemist, Rene Gatefosse researched the use of essential oils in the treatment of physical and psychological conditions. He coined the term aromatherapy for this treatment. Since that time the use of aromatherapy has gained credibility. In France alone it is being used with conventional treatment by a growing number of medical practitioners, who are trained in both traditional medicine and aromatherapy.

Aromatherapy involves the use of the organic essence of aromatic plants for healing the body, mind and spirit. The oils are obtained from the plants by using distillation and solvent extraction. Each oil has its own properties, and oils are often used in conjunction with each other to offer a comprehensive treatment to the client. As some of the oils are contraindicated in certain conditions, aromatherapy should only be administered by a qualified practitioner. Massage can be of great benefit to the client, promoting relaxation and calmness. The combination of massage and aromatherapy can be of particular benefit in substance misuse, allowing the client 'time out' from stress. Aromatherapy is welcomed by most clients attending services.

There is a lack of empirical findings in the nursing literature on the efficacy of aromatherapy to make a claim for its inclusion as part of nursing practice. Research on randomized controlled trials that have been carried out into the therapeutic effect of essential oils used by nurses are documented elsewhere (Valnet

1990; Balacs, 1992; Stevensen, 1994). However, there is no available literature on the use of aromatherapy in the addiction field.

Reflexology

In the UK, reflexology is the third most popular complementary therapy used by nurses (Trevelyan, 1996). In China reflexology is widely used in primary and preventive healthcare (Adamson, 1994). The massage of the feet was documented over 5 000 years ago, when it is thought to have been used as a treatment for both physical and psychological problems. This practice was used by the peoples of ancient China, Japan, Egypt, and North America. Reflexology as we know it today stems from the work developed by Dr William Fitzgerald in the late 1890s. By applying pressure to certain zones, pain relief would be felt in the connected part of the body. This practice, known as zone therapy, was taken a step further to develop a technique known today as reflexology whereby the three zones of the hands, feet or head are massaged to treat physical, psychological and emotional ailments.

Reflexology is one of the many complementary treatments on offer to clients who present with substance misuse problems. The practitioner will work on the feet or hands, feeling for imbalance and energy blockage. These areas will be worked on by using a technique of compression massage, in which the thumbs and fingers are used to apply pressure. The practitioner will remain focused throughout the procedure, allowing the passage of chi. Most clients enjoy the massage element alone, which allows them time out to relax in a quiet and safe environment. On a deeper level reflexology can help to heal physical, psychological and emotional problems.

Complementary therapies in HIV/AIDS

Although this chapter has concentrated on the use of complementary therapies in substance misuse, it is important to mention briefly their use in the clinical management of HIV/AIDS. It is beyond the scope of this chapter to provide a comprehensive exposition on the use of complementary therapies with HIV/AIDS clients. The essential aspect of complementary therapies such as acupuncture, aromatherapy and reflexology is the technique known as therapeutic touch. Clients with HIV and terminal illness are more likely to have increased needs for physical contact to alleviate stress, isolation and rejection. Therapeutic touch can facilitate the nurse–client relationships by increasing empathy and trust thereby allowing more effective interpersonal communications.

Massage as therapy is an acceptable and well-established intervention for clients with HIV/AIDS. The London Lighthouse (1990), Britain's first major residential and support centre for patients affected by HIV and AIDS, not only offers therapies such as massage, reflexology, acupuncture and aromatherapy to their clients but also offers training in complementary therapies.

CONCLUSION

Complementary therapies can be of great value in substance misuse services by increasing the options of care for this client group. Addiction nurses should play a key role in the process of integrating complementary therapies with conventional approaches to care. The advantage of using any of the complementary therapies is that it is more economical compared with the expense of using drugs such as methadone or clonidine. There is no danger of therapeutic addiction. It is important that addiction nurses understand the complexities of complementary therapies and appreciate that formal training is necessary to give adequate knowledge and understanding before incorporating it into their professional practice (Stevensen, 1994). Valid research proving the safety and effectiveness of complementary therapies and the adequate professional and legal regulations are of vital importance. For therapies to become part of the professional nursing practice we must also be prepared to undertake research in order to justify that our actions are based upon knowledge rather than belief (Rankin-Box, 1991).

In 1991, the formation of a special interest group in complementary therapies (RCN) has provided the impetus in the development of guidelines and standards in education and clinical practice. Trevelyan (1996) suggests that complementary therapies are now an important part of nursing but the efficacy of the value of the therapies need be evaluated, and employers need to develop appropriate policies for their use in the NHS. In the immediate future, within the context of nursing, complementary therapies can only serve as adjunctive techniques as part of the total intervention strategies. Addiction nurses interested in the use of complementary therapies should examine its scope, nature and benefits so that these therapies may be offered in caring for substance misusers.

REFERENCES

Adamson, S. (1994) Best Feet Foremost ... reflexology. *Health Visitor*, **67**(2), 61.

Balacs, T. (1992) Dermal crossing. *International Journal of Aromatherapy*, **4**(2), 23–5.

Burke, C. and Sikora, K. (1992) Cancer – the dual approach. *Nursing Times*, **88**(38), 62–6.

Chen, J.Y.P. (1979) *Treatment of cigarette smoking by auricular acupuncture: a report of 184 cases*. Presented at the National Symposia of Acupuncture and Moxibustion and Acupuncture Anaesthesia, January 1–5, 1979, Beijing, China..

Consumers' Association (1995) Healthy choice? *Which?, Report, Consumers' Association*, **11**, 8–13.

Engebretson, J.C. (1992) *Cultural models of healing and health: an ethnography of professional nurses and healers*, The University of Texas, School of Public Health, Houston.

Gates, B. (1994) The use of complementary and alternative therapies in healthcare: a selective review of the literature and discussion of the implications for nurse practitioners and health-care managers. *Journal of Clinical Nursing*, **3**(1), 43–7.

Gomez, E. and Mikhail, A. (1974) Treatment of methadone withdrawal with cerebral electrotherapy (electrosleep). Presented at the annual meeting of the American Psychiatric Association, May 6–10, 1974, Detroit, MI.

Katims, J.J., Ng, L.K.Y. and Lowinson, J.H. (1992) Acupuncture and Transcutaneous Electrical Nerve Stimulation: Afferent Nerve Stimulation (ANS), in *Treatment of Addiction in Substance Abuse: A Comprehensive Textbook*, 2nd edn, (eds J.K. Lowinson, P. Ruiz, R.B. Millman and J.G. Langrod), Williams and Wilkins, Baltimore, pp. 574–83.

London Lighthouse (1990) *Groups, Creative and Complementary Therapies, Activities and Classes for people living with HIV and AIDS*, London Lighthouse, London.

Low, S.A. (1977) Acupuncture and nicotine withdrawal. *Medical Journal of Australia*, **2**, 687.

Malkin, K. (1994) Use of massage in clinical practice. *British Journal of Nursing*, **3**(6), 292–4.

Pfeil, M. (1994) Role of nurses in promoting complementary therapies. *British Journal of Nursing*, **3**(5), 217–19.

Rankin-Box, D. (ed.) (1987) *Complementary Health Therapies. A guide for nurses and the caring professions*. Chapman and Hall, London.

Rankin-Box, D. (1991) Proceed with caution. *Nursing Times*, **87**(45), 34–6.

Smith, M.O. (1979) Acupuncture and natural healing in drug detoxification. *American Journal of Acupuncture*, **7**, 97–107.

Smith, M.O. and Khan, I. (1988) An acupuncture program for the treatment of drug addicted persons. Bulletin of Narcotics, **40**(1), 35–41.

Stevensen, C. (1992) Holistic Power. *Nursing Times*, **88**(38), 68–70.

Stevensen, C. (1994) Aromatherapy: the essentials. RCN Nursing Update, Unit 050. *Nursing Standard*, **9**(9), 3–13.

Thomas, K.J., Carr, J., Westlake, L. and Williams, B.T. (1991) Use of non-orthodox and conventional healthcare in Great Britain. *British Medical Journal*, **302**(6770), 443–7.

Trevelyan, J. (1993) Fringe Benefits. *Nursing Times*, **89**(17), 30–33.

Trevelyan, J. and Booth, B. (1994) *Complementary Medicine for Nurses, Midwives and Health Visitors*, Macmillan, London.

Trevelyan, J. (1996) A true complement? A Nursing Times survey on complementary therapies. *Nursing Times*, **92**(5), 42–3.

UKCC (1992) *Standards for the Administration of Medicines*, UKCC, London.

Valnet, J. (1990) *The Practice of Aromatherapy*, C.W. Daniel, Saffron Walden.

Vickers, A. (1993) *Complementary Medicine and Disability*, Chapman and Hall, London.

Worner, T.M., Zeller, B., Schwarz, H., Zwas, F. and Lyon, D. (1992) Acupuncture fails to improve treatment outcome in alcoholics. *Drug and Alcohol Dependence*, **30**(2), 169–73.

PART THREE

Special populations: issues and interventions

Ethnic minorities and substance misuse

10

G. Hussein Rassool

INTRODUCTION

Race, culture, ethnicity and substance misuse have always been contentious issues from the sociopolitical, economic and health perspectives. Historically, ethnic minorities have been the victims of negative stereotypes with respect to substance misuse. The 1920s saw the 'Birth of the British Drug Underground' and is associated with the popular myth that characterized 'the Chinese population as drug dealers and sexual deviants who preyed upon vulnerable young white women (Kohn, 1992). More recently, the media presentation has resulted in the perception of particular ethnic minorities as being susceptible to the misuse of psychoactive substances. Rastafarians have been associated with cannabis, the Irish with alcohol and Africans have been presented as responsible for the transmission of HIV and AIDS. Nevertheless, these beliefs and stereotypes, with racial undertones, have remained in the popular or collective consciousness of the nation. However, stereotyping masks the full understanding of the state of knowledge regarding the patterns of use, perceptions and health beliefs of ethnic minorities towards the use of psychoactive substances.

The aims of this section are to examine the cultural diversity of ethnic minorities and the nature and extent of substance misuse in these groups. The role of the addiction nurse is also discussed.

CULTURAL DIVERSITY IN ETHNIC GROUPS

The UK is a multicultural society with approximately 6% of the total population, around a total of 3 million people, representing ethnic minorities in England and Wales (OPCS, 1992). Recent classification of ethnic minorities includes Afro-Caribbean (Black African, Black other), Asians (Indian, Pakistani and Bangladeshi), Chinese, Arab, mixed origin, etc. The largest ethnocultural group is

Indians, next the Caribbeans and Pakistanis, followed by Africans, Bangladeshis and Chinese. Most large ethnocultural communities are established in metropolitan geographical areas and reside predominantly in London, the West Midlands, West Yorkshire, and Greater Manchester (Balajaran and Raleigh, 1992;OPCS, 1992). It is apparent that ethnic minorities are a heterogeneous population with diverse cultural entity.

This cultural diversity, with a wide variation in lifestyle, health behaviour, religion and language, has profound effects on their perception and recognition of health problems and ill-health constructed within the paradigm of Western Medicine and the healthcare system (Rassool, 1995). Addiction nurses and other healthcare professionals need to be aware of the existence of ethnic minorities within the community they serve. The practitioners should be able to assess the healthcare needs of the ethnic groups and develop services which take account of linguistic, religious and cultural differences (Department of Health, 1991).

NATURE, EXTENT AND MANAGEMENT OF SUBSTANCE MISUSE

UK research into the use and misuse of psychoactive substances by ethnic minorities has been relatively scarce, although there is extensive North American literature. The differences in the historical, cultural, demographic and nature of ethnocultural groups in the UK and North America mean that direct comparisons cannot be made. In the UK, although there is some literature on the use and misuse of alcohol among Asians and Afro-Caribbeans, the prevalence and incidence in the misuse of illicit drugs are relatively unknown. Only a few regional and local studies have been undertaken to describe epidemiological/behavioural aspects of addiction in ethnic minorities. However, stereotyping tends to mask the full understanding of the state of knowledge regarding the patterns of use and perceptions of health beliefs towards the use of pyschoactive substances.

The substances misused by ethnic minorities are not clearly different from those used by the British majority. However, there seem to be preferences for a certain class or classes of substances and mode of consumption by different ethnic groups which are linked with the historical and cultural characteristics of each ethnic group (Oyefeso and Ghodse, 1993). The studies investigating alcohol-related problems show high levels of alcohol-related morbidity among Asian and Caribbean population (Clarke *et al.*, 1990; Mather and Marjot, 1990). The assumptions that Asian culture is abstemious need to be challenged (Ahmed, 1989). In relation to alcohol use and misuse, Cochrane and Bal (1990) found that 90.5% Asian Muslim men were abstainers and only a very small proportion (0.5%) were heavy drinkers (41+ units per week) in the 41–50 age group. Sikhs had the largest proportion of men drinking over the recommended limits and they were consuming over 40 units of alcohol per week, specially spirit. Older Sikhs drank more compared to the white men of equivalent age. The findings also showed that 11% of Hindus were drinking 21+ units per week, and those born in India were likely to consume more than those born in the UK. Balarajan and Yuen (19864), Haines and Booroff *et al.*, (1987) all produced research evidence which was consistent in showing lower average consumption amongst both Afro-Caribbean men and women than whites. In terms of average units per week, Afro-Caribbean men and women drank significantly less than their white counterparts; Afro-Caribbean men were found to be one third as likely to drink heavily (40+ units per week).

Data obtained from the South West Thames Regional Substance Misuse Database Unit (St George's Hospital Medical School, 1994) showed that, in general, the most commonly reported problem among Indians is alcohol misuse, followed by the use of cannabis. In both the Pakistani and Black groups, the use of opiates is predominant. Among Blacks, the use of opiates is followed by cocaine and cannabis. These observations suggest that the widely held assumptions of the substance-specific cultural stereotypes that Asians and Blacks did not use alcohol and opiates are gradually becoming less tenable. There is also the contention that injecting drug use behaviour is largely uncommon among Asian and Blacks. A recent study in Bradford shows that among the minority of Asian people that used heroin, a percentage did inject (Patel, 1993). This supports the notion of heterogeneity in the pattern of substance misuse in different ethnocultural groups.

There are conflicting reports on the use of tobacco smoking among ethnocultural groups. Some studies show a low prevalence of heavy smoking in Asian and Caribbean men (Waterson and Murray-Lyon, 1989; Balarajan and Yuen, 1986), and others report a high prevalence (McKeigue *et al.*, 1991; 1988). In relation to the transmission of HIV infection, heterosexual intercourse has been the predominant method of HIV infection among those from the Caribbean and African Commonwealth (CDSC, 1992).

Special problems and issues

There is a growing notion and increasing national recognition that our nation's healthcare system is poorly addressing the healthcare needs of ethnic minority communities and that there is inequitable access to services (Alibhai, 1986; Stokes, 1991; Woolett and Dosanjh-Matwala, 1990; Mello, 1992; Murphy and Macleod Clark, 1993). Since its inception, the NHS has been delivering healthcare to its White, culturally homogeneous population (RCN, 1994).

Given the scale of the problem among ethnic groups, under-utilization of substance misuse services by ethnic minorities has been an ongoing concern in the field of addiction. Although, access of ethnic minority groups to substance misuse services have been debated in recent years, many services have been reluctant to acknowledge the need to improve service provision. Many agencies remain mainstream and ethnocentric in their approaches to culturally diverse clients, resulting in poor delivery of service in meeting the health needs of these groups. It has been suggested that institutionalized racism is embedded in the fabric of service provision and delivery. According to Fernando (1993), institutionalized racism 'is not necessarily about people being nasty to one another. It is more about perpetuating traditional attitudes linked to the exercise of power – ignoring or rejecting other people's values and lifestyles, or ideas about illness and health, or about the social use of substances, because we assume our ways are "obviously" much better, more civilized, more advanced, more scientific. It is about unthinking behaviour – or the refusal to think because it is easier and more comfortable not to'.

The low rates of presentation to services by ethno-cultural groups may be due to a multitude of factors that include cultural values' systems, cultural dissonance, education and literacy, previous experience of persecution, communication difficulties, religiocultural prescriptions and discrimination (Oyefeso and Ghodse, 1993; Rassool 1995). Lack of knowledge of service provision and communication difficulties were found as barriers in the utilization of healthcare services (Centre for Mass Communication Research, 1989). It is argued that ethnic groups do not perceive substance misuse services as meeting their needs, and to attend may be conceived either as a threat to themselves or to their self-image. It is acknowledged that there are intrinsic barriers to help-seeking behaviour within cultures. There is evidence to suggest that some members of the Asian population would not want to attend drug services within their community for fear of it becoming known within their own community (Awiah et al., 1992).

Ethnic monitoring and access to services

The health issues raised in *The Health of the Nation* document (Department of Health, 1992) have significant relevance for ethnic minority groups. It has been shown that the underlying aetiology and causation of many conditions is different in ethnic minority populations from that seen in the indigenous population (Department of Health, 1993). In addition, the Chief Medical Officer's report (Calman, 1992) states that in order to meet the healthcare needs of its local population, a health authority's first requirement is to obtain accurate information about the ethnic mix of its populations, its cultural habits and its health status, and take positive steps to eliminate discrimination. Ethnic monitoring of inpatients' admission within the NHS in England, became a mandatory requirement from the 1 April 1995. In the substance misuse field, ethnic monitoring has become a subject of immense importance in order to identify gaps in service provision.

Ethnic monitoring can be defined as 'the determination of the relevant proportion of persons, or behaviour, of different ethnic groups within a specified population' (Oyefeso et al., 1996). It is 'the process of recording ethnic origin, analysing and interpreting the results, and using the information to modify and improve practice' (Karmi, 1996). Oyefeso et al. (1996) suggest that ethnic monitoring allows the evaluation of how accessible different types of services are to different ethnic groups in order that resource allocation, policy and service developments may be more finely tuned to ensure the delivery of an equitable service. However, if the process is used merely to record ethnicity, without a consequent change in health practice, then it may arouse the suspicion that it collects 'race data' for clandestine use (Karmi, 1996). Guidelines on the implementation of ethnic monitoring and collection of ethnic group data are discussed by Karmi and Horton (1992) and the NHS Executive (1994).

In order to improve access to services by ethnic minority population, two main strategies have been advocated by Harrison *et al.*, (1996). Service providers need to consider strategies that include: enhancement of access to mainstream services and the creation of separate agencies run by ethnic minorities workers. Patel (1993) offers a valuable account of how a mainstream service dealing with substance misuse undertook developmental outreach work to widen the access of services to ethnic minority groups. He suggests the following framework:

- outreach work – identify the needs of the community and forge an alliance with key individuals in the local community;
- employ ethnic workers to gain credibility and trust, and to attract ethnic minority clients to the service;
- employment of ethnic minority staff at all levels of organization. Involvement in policy development and decision-making;
- make up of staff team should reflect cultural diversity of the local population;
- education and training in working with ethnic minorities;
- culturally sensitive advertisement. Use of ethnic media such as newspapers and radio programmes.

Nursing and other interventions

The UKCC *Code of Professional Conduct* (1992) points out that 'each registered nurse is accountable for his or her practice, and in the exercise of professional accountability, shall take account of the customs, values and spiritual beliefs of patients/clients'. It is stated that, in order to provide an equitable healthcare service to non-English speaking patients or clients, a bilingual health advocate is necessary (RCN, 1994). Murphy and Clark's (1993) studies demonstrate that there is an urgent need to develop cultural knowledge in nurse education programmes and that nurses need help and support with communication difficulties. Interpreting services and dietary requirements were also found to be inadequate. Accessible information on the health and customs of ethnic minorities are found in Karmi (1996).

Addiction nurses must be aware of their own cultural expectations and not impose these upon clients from different cultures. They need to challenge and confront their own prejudice and negative perception of ethnic minorities and to consider the composition of different ethnic and cultural backgrounds of their patients in order to deliver safe and effective care. Due to the significant differences between the ethnocultural groups in lifestyles, health behaviour, disease patterns and mortality levels, appropriate nursing interventions should be tailored to meet the specific health needs of the individual group.

Patients from different cultural and ethnic backgrounds may present a special challenge to addiction nurses and the multidisciplinary team in the assessment of substance misuse. These difficulties are accentuated because of cultural variations in the presentation of symptoms and where a 'dual diagnosis' – substance misuse and psychiatric disorders – is ascribed. Some ethnocentric nursing interventions are clearly biased towards the dominant culture and mainstream counselling may be inappropriate for some ethnic groups. Many ethnic minorities have very little knowledge or real experience of counselling or the counselling process. A client-centred approach, as advocated by the literature, may not be the type of approach that the client is looking for. On the other hand, the counsellor could be perceived as a figure of authority who would intervene and 'cure' all ills. Finn (1994) has demonstrated the number of approaches that substance misuse counsellors can adopt for increasing their cultural responsiveness to ethnic minority clients thereby improving treatment effectiveness.

There are several issues and problems that have emerged through the practical provision of services to ethnic minorities. These include; religious beliefs, spiritual healing, family pride, destiny, culture, patriarchy, gender issues and perceiving the worker as the prime mover for problem-solving. The provision and exchange of health information and directive counselling may be more appropriate in this context. However, styles and patterns of communication vary widely between the various ethnic minority groups and within each ethnic minority group. It is vital for the counsellor to be aware of how communication is received and interpreted as there are different patterns of intonation for those not having English as their first language (Ahmed, 1988). The format, content and intent of communication needs to be culturally sensitive.

Trans-cultural approach

A transcultural approach may be more appropriate as part of the therapeutic intervention strategies in the management of substance misuse in ethnic minorities. According to Leininger (1988), cross-cultural communication skills may lead to three potential modes of intervention: care oriented towards cultural preservation, cultural negotiation or cultural repatterning. Whether the outcome is cultural preservation, accommodation or change, the goal is that the outcomes of intervention are acceptable, meaningful and satisfying to the client (Leininger, 1988). An aspect of the intervention strategies in managing substance misuse is the use of transcultural counselling. D'Ardenne and Mahtani (1989) stated that 'transcultural counselling is not about being an expert or any given culture but a way of thinking about clients where culture is acknowledged and valued'.

Addiction nurses adopting a transcultural approach to counselling (Daniels, 1993) will need to have the following:

- knowledge of the psychosocial and psychological effects of drugs and their potential for harm;
- knowledge of the sociocultural context, with specific reference to community from which the client comes, as well as linguistic accessibility where relevant;

- assessment skills with appropriate sensitivity to the client's sociocultural and individual needs;
- access to a variety of conceptual models. Ability to apply the models in a variety of cultural settings;
- skills in applying cross-cultural and anti-racist perspectives to their work.
- skills in interventions aimed at harm-reduction and harm-minimization. Ability to effect change in a cultural context, taking into account the individual's constructs and beliefs.

CONCLUSION

Substance misuse and addiction in ethnic minorities in the UK need to be considered in the context of sociopolitical perspectives and the permeation of racism. The issues related to working with substance misusers from ethnic minorities include language, culture, patriarchy, gender issues, religious beliefs, family pride, health beliefs, stigma, confidentiality, oppression and racism. To work effectively with this client group does not require one to become an expert in all ethnocultural groups but to have cultural flexibility, acceptance and understanding; and to perceive the patient or client as an individual (Rassool, 1995). What is considered essential is to develop an openness to cultural diversity to the relativity of our own beliefs, values and culture. There is an urgent need to prepare addiction nurses and other healthcare professionals for race issues to enable them to work in a culturally sensitive manner.

REFERENCES

Ahmed, N. (1988) *Service provisions for Ethnic Minority Problem Drinkers from an Asian Background*, Southall Alcohol Advisory Service, Middlesex.

Ahmed, N. (1989) *Service provisions for Ethnic Minority Problem Drinkers from an Asian Background*, Proceedings of the 35th International Congress on Alcoholism and Drug Dependency, Oslo, pp. 36–43.

Alibhai, Y. (1986) Culture Shocks. *New Society*, **78**, 11.

Awiah, J., Butt, S. and Dorn, N. (1992) *Race, Gender and Drug Services*, Institute for the Study of Drug Dependence, London.

Balarajan, R. and Yuen, P. (1986) British smoking and drinking habits: variations by country of birth. *Community Medicine*, **8**(3), 237–39.

Balarajan, R. and Soni Raleigh, V. (1992) The ethnic populations of England and Wales: the 1991 census. *Health Trends*, **24**(4), 113–16.

Calman, K.C. (1992) *On the State of the Public Health 1991: The Annual Report of the Chief Medical Officer of the Department of Health for the year 1991*, HMSO, London.

Centre for Mass Communication Research (1989) *Evaluation of the Asian Mother and Baby Campaign*, University of Leicester, Leicester.

Clarke, M., Ahmed, N., Romaniuk, H., Marjot, D.H. and Murray-Lyon, I.M. (1990) Ethnic differences in the consequences of alcohol misuse. *Alcohol and Alcoholism*, **25**(1), 9–11.

Cochrane, R. and Bal, S.S. (1990) The drinking patterns of Sikh, Hindu, Muslim and White men in the West Midlands: a community survey. *British Journal of Addiction*, **85**(6), 759–69.

Communicable Disease Surveillance Centre (1992) *AIDS/HIV Quarterly Surveillance Tables*, 28.

D'Ardenne, P. and Mahtani, A. (1989) *Transcultural Counselling in Action*, Sage, London.

Daniels, O. (1993) Trans-Cultural Therapy for Substance Problems, in *Race Culture and Substance Problems* (ed. L. Harrison) Department of Social Policy and Professional Studies, The University of Hull, Hull.

Department of Health (1991) *The Patient's Charter* HMSO, London.

Department of Health (1992) *The Health of the Nation. A Strategy for Health in England*, HMSO, London.

Department of Health (1993) *The Health of the Nation. Ethnicity and Health*, HMSO, London.

Fernando, S. (1993) Race, Culture and Substance Problems, in *Race Culture and Substance Problems* (ed. L. Harrison) Department of Social Policy and Professional Studies, The University of Hull, Hull.

Finn, P. (1994) Addressing the needs of cultural minorities in drug treatment. *Journal of Substance Abuse Treatment*, **11**(4), 325–27.

Haines, A.P., Booroff, A., *et al.* (1987) Blood pressure, smoking, obesity and alcohol consumption in black and white patients in general practice. *Journal of Human Hypertension*, **1**(1), 39–46.

Harrison, L., Harrison, M. and Adebowale, V. (1996) Drinking problems among Black communities, in *Alcohol Problems in the Community* (ed. L. Harrison), Routledge, London, pp. 223–40.

Karmi, G. and Horton, C. (1992) *Guidelines for the implementation of Ethnic Monitoring. The Health and Ethnicity Programme*, NE and NW Thames Regional Health Authorities, London.

Karmi, G. (1996) *The Ethnic Health Handbook: A factfile for health care professionals*, Blackwell Science, Oxford.

Kohn, M. (1992) *Dope Girls: The Birth of the British Drug Underground*, Lawrence and Wishart, London.

Leininger, M.M. (1988) Leininger's theory of nursing: Cultural care diversity and Universality. *Nursing Science Quarterly*, **1**(4), 152–60.

Mather, H.M. and Marjot, D.H. (1990) Alcohol-related admissions to a psychiatric hospital: a comparison of Asians and Europeans. *British Journal of Addiction*, **84**(3), 327–29.

Mello, M. (1992) Plugging the gap – diabetes – UK's ethnic minorities – provision for them is limited and reflects wider racial issues. *Nursing Times*, **88**(43), 34–6.

McKeigue, P.M., Shah, B. and Marmot, M.G. (1991) Relation of central obesity and insulin resistance with high diabetes prevalence and cardiovascular risk in South Asians. *Lancet*, **337**(8738), 382–86.

McKeigue, P.M., Marmot, M.G., Syndercombe Court, Y.D., *et al.* (1988) Diabetes, hyperinsulinaemia, and coronary risk factors in Bangladeshis in East London. *British Heart Journal*, **60**(5), 390–96.

Murphy, K. and Macleod Clark, J. (1993) Nurses' experiences of caring for ethnic-minority clients. *Journal of Advanced Nursing*, **18**(3), 442–50.

National Health Service Executive (1994) *Collecting Ethnic Group Data for Admitted Patient Care*, Department of Health, London.

Office of Population Censuses and Surveys (1992) *1991 Census: Outline statistics for England and Wales*: National Monitor CEN 91 CM 58, HMSO, London.

Oyefeso, A. and Ghodse, A.H. (1993) Addictive Behaviour, in *Ethnic Minorities*. Paper presented at the National Workshop on Assessing the Health Needs of People from Ethnic Minorities, London.

Oyefeso, A., Jones, M. and Ghodse, A.H. (1996) Ethnic monitoring in specialist drug services: a population-based analysis. *Journal of Substance Misuse*, **1**(2), 91–96

Owen, D. (1994) Spatial variations in ethnic minority group populations in Great Britain. *Population Trends*, **78**(23–33), winter.

Patel, K. (1993) Ethnic Minority access to services, in *Race, Culture and Substance Problems* (ed. L. Harrison), Department of Social Policy and Professional Studies. University of Hull.

Rassool, G.H. (1995) The Health Status and Health Care of Ethno-Cultural Minorities in the United Kingdom: An Agenda for Action. *Journal of Advanced Nursing*, **21**(2), 199–201.

Royal College of Nursing (1994) *Black and ethnic minority patients and clients: meeting needs*: Nursing Update, Learning Unit 032, RCN, London.

Stokes, G. (1991) A transcultural nurse is about. *Senior Nurse*, **11**(1), 40–2.

Waterson, E.J. and Murray-Lyon, I.M. (1989) Alcohol, smoking and pregnancy: some observations on ethnic minorities in the United kingdom. *British Journal of Addiction*, **84**(3), 323–25.

Woollett, A. and Dosanjh-Matwala, N. (1990) Postnatal care: the attitudes and experiences of Asians women in East London. *Midwifery*, **6**(4), 178–84.

United Kingdom Central Council for Nursing, Midwifery and Health Visiting (1992) *Code of Professional Conduct*, 3rd edn. UKCC, London.

11

Women and substance misuse

Kris Dominy

INTRODUCTION

In the UK there are a considerable number of services specifically geared towards meeting the healthcare needs of female substance misusers. However, service provision in the UK appears to be failing to attract women or to offer appropriate responses (DAWN, 1994), and as a group women face formidable barriers to treatment. Healthcare professionals are becoming increasingly aware that women have different and quite specific needs to men and recognize that there is a pressing need to address the issue of how best these needs could be met. The needs of women are different to men in relation to physiological and biological make up. Issues, such as childbearing, motherhood, society's gender roles, expectations and psychological make up, all contribute to a different pathway into addiction. Consequently, the problems, conflicts and issues tend to mount once addicted. Recent information bears out the fact that both drug and alcohol use among women is rising. Therefore, attention must be paid to the diversity of needs of this client group. Addiction nursing is pivotal in the care of substance misusers as these clients are becoming increasingly prevalent throughout all areas of nursing care.

The aims of this chapter will focus on a range of substances including alcohol, although it should be pointed out that the issue of women and substance misuse alone, is vast and requires specific attention which is not possible here. This chapter does not aim to be prescriptive and the objective is to provide an outline of some of the major difficulties in dealing with this client group.

NATURE AND EXTENT OF SUBSTANCE MISUSE

While there is data available from the Home Office regarding prevalence rates of addicted women, it is important to bear in mind however that such data are likely to underestimate the size of the problem. Women are less likely to admit to using drugs when there are related childcare issues. The most recent data from the Home Office suggest that for every notified woman addict there are three men. This is an increase from the recent the figure of 1:4. Each year since 1988, the age of female addicts, whether new or re-notified, has become lower. The female average age for new addicts is lower than the total average age. Since 1989 there has been an increase each year in notified female addicts (1989 − 1 687 females; 1993 − 2 580 females). The average age being 28.2 − 28.8. (ISDD, 1994).

The most recent research into the differences between male and female drug users (Powis *et al.*, 1996) found that of the women questioned 45% used cocaine and 38% heroin. Women were more likely to chase than inject heroin but female injectors tended to be younger than their male counterparts and have higher levels of dependence. The results of this study also point to the fact that there is a clear disparity in the numbers of women using substances who have no contact with any form of treatment with the numbers usually found in treatment populations.

Statistics from the new General Household Survey show that since 1984 the proportion of women drinking at risky or dangerous levels has steadily risen. The highest proportion of women drinking above recommended limits occurs in the 'single' category, and this behaviour is clearly related to the socioeconomic grouping of 'professional' and 'employer/manager' women. There are, however, a number of issues that are of particular concern with regard to female substance misusers and it is on these that attention must be directed. One of the most prominent of these concerns is the misuse of tranquillizers either prescribed or illicitly acquired. Department of Health statistics (1991) showed that 21 million prescriptions for hypnotics, sedatives and tranquillizers were issued, the vast majority of these being for benzodiazepines. With many of these being repeat prescriptions to women clients not seen by their GP, it is reasonable to infer that this is a significant contributor to substance misuse difficulties experienced by women.

THE LIFESTYLES OF WOMEN DRUG USERS

It is imperative that the full range of life variables are taken into account when comparing the differences between male and female substance users and this section is an attempt to highlight some of the more significant substance related issues that are specific to women. The first involves the type of substances and the range of reasons for their use. For example, many women have tranquillizers prescribed by their GP and their use is problematic but not likely to be brought to the attention of addiction services. Around 12 million prescriptions for tranquillizers are issued by GPs in this country per annum frequently resulting in a dependence that may not provide the tabloid images of intravenous opiate use but which, nonetheless, is problematic.

This may be indicative of one of the main differences in both pattern and profile of substance use between sexes. Female drug use may less frequently be characterized by binge use resulting in aggressive and antisocial behaviour but this merely reflects disparities in patterns of use rather than prevalence. As with female alcohol users, female drug users may make less noise without necessarily having less of a problem. This is compatible with the hypothesis that the substance activity of women may frequently have as its foundation not the desire for hedonistic effect associated with male substance activity but a number of specific objectives. These may include the use of alcohol or tranquillizers as a palliative for domestic violence, the use of opiates and alcohol to overcome the stigma of engaging in paid sex or the use of stimulants, in particular amphetamines, to cope with the everyday rigours of family life, to name but three.

These differences may also result from the diversity of routes into a substance misuse career. Women are more likely to commence use as consequence of the activities of their sexual partners than their peer groups. Also the route into illicit substance misuse may be initiated by prescriptions for pain relief, neurotic illness or depression or through the use of slimming tablets. These differences in drug history may well indicate a differing approach to the problem and its resolution, one which is sensitive to the differing roles and lifestyles of female drug users from that of their male counterparts. Thus, the frequently clandestine nature of female substance activity, whether this takes the form of the abuse of prescribed drugs or the refusal of many women to enter drug agencies is a manifestation of the subjugated status of women generally in society and, in particular, the specific stigma that attaches itself to female drug users. For this reason, treatment services must attempt to make provision for the particular needs of female drug users. It is important to reject the social stereotypes of female substances use and to break the cycle of subjugation, humiliation and mistrust that are daily aspects of female substance use and, sadly, treatment.

Specific issues

Pregnancy

The majority of women who misuse drugs and alcohol are of childbearing age, and many come from disadvantaged unhealthy environments, lacking economic and social support. However, due to fear of statutory authority combined with chaotic life styles many female substance misusers who are pregnant fail to attend antenatal or GP services. Consequently, one of the first aims of treatment would be to identify and attract female substance misusers to services, by providing a non-judgemental, 'user-friendly' and comprehensive approach to care which enables access to necessary and appropriate services. The female substance misuser needs to be in regular contact with both antenatal and drug counselling services in order for the complexity of needs to be addressed. The client herself requires services, support and appropriate counselling to make the decision whether to stabilize her current drug use or begin the process of detoxifying. Decisions will be necessary about whether to reduce all 'street' drugs and replace with oral drugs, and whether to receive care on an in-patient or community basis. Research shows that the safest possible time to detoxify from substances of dependence is after the 14th week and before the 28th week of pregnancy in order to minimize the risk of miscarriage in the first trimester, or precipitative premature labour and foetal distress in the last trimester (National Institute on Drug Abuse, 1985).

A detoxification regimen, for example in the case of opiate dependence, requires appropriate medical supervision and should be conducted at a comfortable pace for both the mother and unborn child. On an inpatient basis it is easier to monitor the detoxification regimen and follow an assessment of need; a period of 21 days appears to be a suitable period of time. Obviously during this time the woman needs to establish and maintain her contact with the antenatal clinic and hospital where her delivery will take place. The psychological issues surrounding pregnancy are varied but may include the following.

- Whether the pregnancy was planned or not? The difficult question of whether the baby is wanted if the pregnancy is unplanned may arise and must be dealt with sensitively and in a nonjudgmental approach.
- Social services involvement may anger the mother. She could feel that she is not being given a chance to prove herself and that the control of her pregnancy is being taken away from her. Antenatal planning meetings are a great source of stress and suspicion for both the mother and father, and support, advice and information is needed during this process. The woman and her partner should be encouraged to enter into constructive dialogue with their social worker.
- If the woman is on her own, this may be from personal choice, the father of the child not wanting to be part of the process or not knowing who the father is. Whatever the reason the woman should be encouraged to establish a support network so that she is not isolated following the birth of her baby.
- Preparation for motherhood – the use of illicit drugs prevents certain aspects of emotional and psychological development and growth, and the process of preparation for motherhood does not escape this. The role of the nurse is to facilitate the woman's progress through this process in an attempt to enable her to prepare herself. The woman must be reminded that she needs to consider the consequences of her actions on her unborn child but this must not appear to be used as a weapon to cause guilt, leading to resentment of the child. Similarly, the issue of termination may be reviewed during this period and the worker needs training in abortion counselling to tackle this issue satisfactorily or alternatively should refer the woman appropriately.
- If the female substance misuser is infected with HIV she would be faced with complex decisions regarding the pregnancy. The ACMD report (1988) advocates that women who are HIV positive should avoid becoming pregnant, but once pregnant it does not recommend termination in all HIV infected women as this may result in women not coming forward for antenatal care. Research by Johnstone et al. (1990) also highlights the special considerations that women should take into account, such as whether to continue or to terminate a pregnancy.

The ACMD perspective is that termination should be offered as an option but not forced upon the woman. Counselling should be made available in order to assist the woman to make the right decision for her particular circumstances. In the area of HIV the risk of pregnancy to mother and child is still uncertain. Professionals who come into contact with this group of women should keep up-to-date with current knowledge and treatment in order to remain responsive, and they should have the best available information for the client.

It is important to remember that substance misuse, be that drugs or alcohol, is only one aspect of the range of problems the pregnant woman has to face. A holistic approach within a multidisciplinary setting should be adopted which aims to optimize the physical, emotional and practical care the woman can be offered.

Prostitution

The link between drug, alcohol use and prostitution is well established and there are a number of possible reasons for these links. One is that prostitution is widely used by some women as a means of financing their drug habit – the link being economic. Another is that drugs or alcohol may be used as a means of coping with having to be a prostitute – the link being psychological or emotional. A further link may be that of sexual exploitation by a violent partner who may or may not be using drugs or alcohol themselves but may use the woman's prostitution for financial gain or to support their habit. It is also possible for the drug or alcohol use and prostitution to develop independently.

In a recent study of sexual behaviour and its relationship to drug taking among prostitutes in South London (Gossop *et al.*, 1994) 59% of the women questioned said that one of the main reasons for working as a prostitute was to pay for drugs, and 55% reported having given sex for drugs on at least one occasion. Most often this was with a dealer, and the drugs most often exchanged were heroin and cocaine.

There are a number of issues of concern when addressing the needs of this group of women. Clearly, the risk of contracting HIV, hepatitis B or C are increased. In the study mentioned above (Gossop *et al.*, 1994) the women questioned were more willing to have unsafe sex if the price was right or if they knew the client well. Obviously, this carries high risk for both the women and the clients involved. The women involved reported rarely or never using condoms with their regular partners, some of whom were injecting drug users. The risks are clearly multiplied with this group of women who are engaging in a variety of unsafe drug injecting practices and many women had shared injecting equipment.

Alcohol consumption

Many women in this group reported regularly drinking before seeing clients in order to help them cope with working as a prostitute. Most were drinking at levels which exceeded recommended safe limits for women and some were drinking at levels which are likely to cause physical harm. Recent changes in the government's recommendations for safe drinking limits to 21 units per week for women have caused concern as there are many women drinking in excess of previous limits who may be encouraged to further increase their alcohol consumption. Gossop *et al.* (1994) identified that women who worked as prostitutes to finance their drug habit were more severely dependent on their drug of choice, e.g. heroin. In addition, by using the drugs this included all the identified health hazards of drug misuse e.g. poor health, nutritional shortfall, aggravated infections, infected injection sites, abscesses, risk of deep vein thrombosis and so on in addition to the risk to health from prostitution itself.

Sex and sexuality

The issues surrounding sex and sexuality play a major part in understanding the process of working with female drug users and the context and history of their substance activity. As Hser *et al.* (1987) point out women are more likely to be introduced to drug use by a sexual partner than are men, and Powis *et al.* (1995) concluded that many women are given their first injection by a sexual partner. This association between the drug activity of women and their primary relationship recurs throughout the literature with a cross-section claiming that women drug users are more likely than men to have drug using sexual partners (Gossop *et al.* 1994), to have their drug use supported by a partner (Anglin *et al.* 1987) and to share injecting equipment with a sexual partner (Barnard, 1993).

The implication of these research findings is that for many women both the initiation and continuation of both substance use in general and drug injection in particular is associated with their primary sexual relationship. This may lead them to a distorted understanding of love, men, intimacy, sexuality, tenderness and all the other components of normal relationship development. The problems associated with the joint development of a relationship and substance dependence may make the relationship unhealthy. This often results in women presenting at services that may be viewed with mistrust and suspicion with a history of damaging and exploitative relationships with male drug users.

This is exacerbated by the frequently problematic backgrounds of many female substance users who, according to Stanton (1980), are likely to have experienced conflict and unhappiness in their family of origin, substance misuse by parents or siblings and frequent and prolonged separation from parents. Similarly, Rohsenow *et al.*, (1988) reports child sexual abuse in a substantial subgroup of female addicts. Thus, there would appear to be two issues which may be more prominent for female drug users and which are likely to influence treatment outcomes – a history of family problems possibly culminating in some form of sexual abuse and the association between substance misuse and current personal circumstances. If it is reasonable to infer, as the evidence suggests, that the aetiology and maintenance of female substance problems have a more powerful social and interpersonal foundation than those of men then the issues of female sexuality and its impact on substance activity must be addressed while the woman is in treatment. Although it is a generally held view that women do less well in treatment services when they have substance abusing partners.

The problem may often be that what women fear most is being alone and that the solution to this is to move from one harmful relationship to another, often with male substance users. Clearly, few relationships can succeed when both partners have dependency issues and this may lead to a cycle of short and damaging relationships for the women involved, a situation exacerbated when pregnancy or childrearing issues are involved. The fact that alcohol and drug use are often contributory factors to both sexual abuse and domestic violence can only complicate the situation further and may contribute to women's feelings of low esteem, worthlessness, guilt and depression which may result in significant mental health problems.

Faced with such a complicated and self-perpetuating problem treatment services must be realistic in their goals and focus on providing a safe and nonjudgemental environment where the woman can address her situation openly and honestly. The emphasis should be on enabling the woman to gain insight into the patterns of behaviour she is engaged in and to facilitate any decisions she makes to change. This process may be punctuated with anxiety, fear and pain as the reality of her situation becomes more clear. The issue of co-dependence is difficult for many women to understand, far less to escape from. Although there is little evidence to support the view that many addiction nurses feel that relationships formed during drug using periods have no future, it is generally accepted that time apart to re-evaluate the relationship is needed. The pressure that a partner can place on a woman is enormous and she must be given the support and time to make the right decision for her, whatever that decision may be.

SERVICE PROVISION

In order for services to offer effective treatment, consideration must be given to the differences between male and female substance misusers. There is a suggestion that female substance misusers are not being attracted into treatment services in the same proportions as their male counterparts. Women fear that by virtue of being addicted to illicit drugs, they are perceived as 'unfit' mothers and that social services will remove their children. The ACMD report (1989) addressed this issue emphasizing that social service departments must make it known that drug misuse is in itself not a reason to remove a child from its parents. However, the fear of authority continues and drug users represent a cohort particularly suspicious of statutory authority.

The National Addiction Centre recently conducted a consumer audit on clients' satisfaction with treatment services. Many of the women felt dissatisfied with service provision in a number of areas:

- models of treatment were perceived as catering for the needs of male drug users;
- services were seen as male dominated in terms of staff as well as clients;
- services are seen as having either poor or no childcare facilities;
- women fear that their children will be taken into care if they enter treatment.

In support of this many women reported that being separated from their children detered them from entering residential treatment or had caused them to leave treatment prematurely. Other criticisms included the view that services are too male dominated, with the consequence that women feel too intimidated to speak freely in groups and often have to put up with macho behaviour which is often sexist and crude. The choice is either become 'one of the boys' or be seen as a killjoy. Women also do not wish to be identified as drug users, as this may conflict with the ideal of the stereotypical female role (Barnard, 1993).

Matching treatment to client needs

The aim of treatment would be to attract women into services and to maintain contact. There have been debates on whether women-only services are the solution to the problem. However, the women asked in the service audit mentioned above stated that they would prefer women's sessions in existing services rather than separate services for women. Considering the current economic and political climate where services are being reduced rather than expanded, service providers should consider the following points when either planning to develop services or reviewing current services.

- Raising consciousness of the need to find realistic solutions for women in those involved in both the purchasing of services and the management of services.
- Developing skilled workers who have awareness and insight into the problems and difficulties facing women who abuse substances.
- Establishing partnership relationships with other affiliated providers, i.e. antenatal clinics, GP services, sexually transmitted disease (STD) or GUM clinics.
- Women should be able to participate in women only groups which include a female group facilitator.
- In a mixed group setting, if at all possible, one of the group facilitators should be female.
- In a residential setting there should be adequate separation between male and female sleeping accommodation, washing and changing facilities.
- Flexible opening times that take childcare issues into account.
- The provision of a service environment where women feel safe, protected and understood when they attend.
- An assessment of the consequences of many women's history of dependence on men as well as substances resulting in a need for practical help in education, housing, employment.
- Treatment facilities that allow access to children and which have adequately

trained staff to look after them when the woman is participating in the service programme.

Interventions

The primary aims of treatment of this group is to engage them in some sort of treatment service e.g. drug clinics, street agency, needle exchange, community drug team. It is vital to provide a nonjudgmental service that preserves their dignity. Women who prostitute themselves to finance their drug habits are seen as 'the lowest of the low' to other drug users, particularly their male counterparts, and service providers must in no way mirror any of these attitudes. At times, inappropriate sexually disinhibited behaviour can manifest itself in flirtations and sexually aggressive forms that may be threatening to both clients and staff (female as well as male members). This must be dealt with tactfully but firmly with the emphasis on preserving the client's dignity.

Contact with treatment services offers a valuable opportunity for the provision of condoms as well as injecting equipment. This time must also be used to provide health counselling, risk-reduction and harm-minimization counselling. Health monitoring can also be carried out and if necessary referral to a GUM/STD Clinic. As many women report prostituting to finance their drug habits, it may be appropriate to consider substituting oral drugs as a means of reducing the associated risks of injecting street drugs.

The overall aim of treatment is to work with the needs of the woman as she perceives them and to use that as a foundation for developing strategies towards lifestyle change and attitudinal shifts. This can only be achieved in an environment in which the woman feels accepted, supported and valued and in which sufficient flexibility is offered to encourage her participation in the ownership of the treatment context.

CONCLUSION

As the numbers of women using drugs and alcohol increase, attention must be directed to the specific needs of this client group. Many current services remain biased towards the needs of male substance misusers, whose profile of substance use career and route into substance misuse may be different from that of their female counterparts. The majority of women who misuse drugs and alcohol are of childbearing age and so the issue of care of the pregnant drug user is of vital importance when planning service provision. Women often fear that their children will be taken into care if their drug use become known. Many services have limited childcare facilities and this may prevent some women from presenting to services.

The message of harm minimization has still not reached many femals drug-using prostitutes who may be reluctant to use condoms with well-known clients or if the price is right. Women prefer to use condoms with clients but feel unable to do so on occasions. Many women resort to prostitution to fund their drug use and recent research points to alcohol consumption in excess of recommended levels in this group of women, yet this is only one area of concern when dealing with women's sexuality and substance use.

Bearing all of the issues raised above, it is not difficult to understand that there are health needs that relate only to women. Services should work towards providing fair and equal access to treatment options which meet the needs of both men and women instead of covering the middle ground which essentially disadvantages and dilutes what is available for both groups. Care and treatment offered must be individually tailored if needs are to be met and the planned outcomes are to be successful. It is imperative that treatment services challenge the subjugated and disempowered status of women drug users and aim to deal with the specific difficulties associated with female drug users

REFERENCES

Advisory Council on the Misuse of Drugs (1988) *AIDS and Drug Misuse Part 1*, HMSO, London.

Advisory Council on the Misuse of Drugs (1989) *AIDS and Drug Misuse Part 1*, HMSO, London.

Anglin, D., Hser, Y. and McGothlin W. (1987) Sex differences in addict careers. 2 Becoming addicted. *American Journal of Drug and Alcohol Abuse*, **13**(3), 253–80.

Barnard, M. (1993) Needle sharing in context : patterns of sharing among men and women injectors and HIV risk. *Addiction*, **88**(6), 805–12.

DAWN (Drugs and Alcohol Women's Network) (1994) *When a Crèche is not Enough. A Survey of Drug and Alcohol Services for Women. Drugs and Alcohol Women's Network*, GLAAS, London.

Department of Health (1991) *Health and personal social services statistics for England*, HMSO, London.

Institute for the Study of Drug Dependence (1994) *Drug Misuse in Britain*, ISDD, London.

Gossop, M., Powis, B., Griffiths, P. and Strang, J. (1994) Sexual behaviour and its relationship to drug taking amongst prostitutes in South London. *Addiction*, **89**(8), 961–70.

Hser, Y., Anglin, D. and Booth, M. (1987) Sex differences in addict careers: 3 Addiction. *American Journal of Drug and Alcohol Abuse*, **13**(1–2), 231–51.

Johnstone, F.D., Brettle, R.P., Mac Cullum, R., *et al.* (1990) Women's knowledge of their antibody state: its effects on their decision whether to continue pregnancy. *British Medical Journal*, **300**(6716), 23–4.

National Institute on Drug Abuse (1985) *Drug dependence in pregnancy : clinical management of mother and child*, National Institute on Drug Abuse, Rockville, M.D, pp. 37.

Powis, B., Griffiths, P., Gossop, M. and Strang, J. The differences between male and female drug users – community samples of Heroin and Cocaine users compared. *Journal of Substance Use and Misuse*, **31**(5), 519–43.

Rohsenow, E.J., Corbett, R. and Devine, D. (1988) Molested as children : a hidden contribution to substance abuse? *Journal of Substance Abuse Treatment*, **5**(Suppl.), 13–8.

Stanton, D.C. (1980) A family theory of drug abuse, in *Theories of drug abuse: selected contemporary perspectives* (eds D. Lettieri and M. Sayers *et al.*), NIDA Research Monograph, Rockville, M.D, pp. 147–57.

Substance misuse in the elderly population

12

Mike Gafoor

INTRODUCTION

Substance misuse among the elderly population has received only scant attention in the UK and with the proportion of people over the age of 65 predicted to increase from 20.8% to 26% by the middle of the next century (OPCS, 1987) the need for effective prevention and treatment strategies warrants urgent consideration by healthcare providers. Both clinicians and researchers have so far tended to focus on younger substance misusers possibly as a result of Winick's (1962) 'maturing out' hypothesis which suggests that some addicts may simply 'burn out' of their addiction or that they do not grow old because they die early. Research carried out recently by McInnes and Powell (1994) indicates that only one quarter of elderly substance misusers admitted to hospital is identified by medical staff and of these only 10% were referred to drug and alcohol services.

There are several reasons why healthcare professionals may fail to identify or respond to a drug or alcohol problem in an old person. Many of the routine screening tests carried out in younger age groups for employment and insurance purposes are not replicated in elderly patients. Even when symptoms of substance misuse are present, these may be attributed to ageing. The patient may also be embarrassed about their substance misuse and conceal the true extent of their problem from healthcare workers. Also family, friends and professionals may deny the existence of the problem, in the misguided belief that they would be taking away the elderly person's only source of pleasure or that nothing can really be done about changing lifelong habits.

This chapter will examine the nature and extent of substance misuse in the elderly population and describe some of the special features and problems associated with this group. The role of the addiction nurse in relation to prevention and treatment of substance misuse in the elderly client will also be discussed.

NATURE AND EXTENT

Research in the UK has shown prevalence rates of alcohol misuse in people over the age of 60 to be 9–13% (Malcolm, 1984) in community surveys, with substantially higher rates found among hospitalized samples (Bridgewater *et al.*, 1987; Bristow and Clare, 1992). Overall it is estimated that between 5% and 12% of men and 1–2% of women in their 60s are problem drinkers (Atkinson,1984).

Elderly alcohol abusers tend to fall into two categories. The first group, is comprised of those drinkers who have had a long history of alcohol abuse and have continued this pattern of drinking into old age. They are also known as early onset alcoholics and constitute up to two-thirds of all elderly alcohol abusers. The second or late onset group are those people who began to abuse alcohol at a later age as a maladaptive response to stressful life events such as bereavement, retirement and loneliness. It has been suggested that up to one-half of elderly alcoholics experience the onset of problem drinking in middle or late life and that more favourable treatment outcomes are achieved with this group (Liberto *et al.*, 1992). Also elderly persons with lower incomes tend to consume less alcohol than those with higher incomes.

The use of illegal substances among the elderly is rare, and problems relating to drug misuse are generally associated with the widespread use of prescribed and 'over the counter' medication. Elderly people receive three times more prescribed medication than the general population (Warren *et al.*, 1985) and psychotropic drugs such as hypnotic sedatives, tranquillizers, anxiolytics and antidepressants are frequently prescribed to older people (Skegg,1979; Jones *et al.*, 1980). It has also been found that the use of pyschotropic medication was more common among older widowed females who tended to have higher levels of psychopathology and were more likely to suffer from symptoms such as confusion, lack of energy, nausea and insomnia (Jones, 1992).

Special problems

The elderly are more susceptible to the effects of chemical substances due to physiological changes associated with the ageing process. Reduction of lean body mass, together with decreased hepatic and renal function result in slowed metabolic breakdown and elimination of drugs. An elderly person will have a higher blood alcohol concentration than a younger person after a standard dose of alcohol. Also neurological changes can lead to impaired cognition and elderly patients experience twice the incidence of paradoxical adverse effects such as ataxia, irritability, hallucinations and nightmares (Caird and Scott, 1986). Substance misuse in the elderly can lead to a variety of conditions including hypothermia, poor hygiene and self neglect, osteoporosis, insomnia, depression, dementia and peripheral neuropathy.

The use of psychotropic medication and in particular benzodiazepines has been associated with an increase in the likelihood of accidents, falls and fractures

(Campbell, 1991; Cooper, 1994). Furthermore, drug-related problems among elderly patients may account for 30–50% of admissions to hospitals and nursing homes (Cooper,1990) and alcohol is a major factor in the development of depression and dementia in the elderly (Saunders *et al.*, 1991). Suicide has also been associated with substance misuse in old age and Wittington (1983) found that barbiturates were most commonly used drugs in suicides among the over 65 group.

Summary of problems

The problems of substance misuse in the elderly can be summarized:

- poor hygiene, self-neglect, hypothermia, chest infections;
- peripheral neuropathy, osteoporosis, cirrhosis;
- accidents, falls, fractures;
- depression, anxiety, insomnia, confusion;
- cognitive impairment, dementia, suicide.

Case vignette

Jean is a 78-year-old widow who has been living on her own in sheltered accommodation since the death of her husband two years ago. She had previously nursed him for over a year after he suffered a stroke. Jean was referred to the local community drug team (CDT) by her GP who was called to see her after she had suffered from yet another fall while intoxicated. Jean had been referred on two previous occasions but failed to answer the door when the CPN arrived. Arrangements were made this time for Jean's daughter to accompany the nurse at the next appointment. Jean described a three year history of alcohol consumption that had increased to half a bottle of whiskey a day since her husband's death. This was being bought for her by a home-help who visited twice a week. At the interview, Jean was alcohol free and was showing objective signs of alcohol withdrawal. She was physically weak and complained of poor appetite and insomnia.

Jean was detoxified from alcohol in hospital with a lorazepam regime and her physical condition improved with the use of vitamin B supplements and build-up drinks. She cited loneliness as the main reason for her drinking and felt no-one cared. She did not want to be a 'burden' to her daughter and became increasingly isolated for fear of being mugged in the streets. Following her discharge from hospital, Jean attended a day centre for the elderly and agreed to taking daily antabuse tablets. Her daughter visited at weekends and took her on outings. The home-help was persuaded not to purchase any further alcohol for Jean who remains abstinent from alcohol.

Nursing interventions

Addiction nurses have an important role in the prevention, treatment and rehabilitation of elderly people with substance misuse problems. For the majority of clients it is neither appropriate nor necessary for them to be treated by a specialist drugs and alcohol service. The primary role of the addiction nurse should be as a specialist resource for healthcare workers involved with this client group, especially those working in the community, in nursing homes and in general hospitals. This would involve providing health advice and information on the adverse physical, social and psychological effects of drug and alcohol misuse in old people as well as the teaching of assessment skills that will help with the early identification of those clients at risk.

In addition, GPs should be advised as to the risks associated with incorrect dosage and unnecessarily long-term prescribing of psychotropic medication. The annual screening programme for the over 75s provides an ideal opportunity for GPs to identify substance misuse problems and to educate their patients. Similarly both clients and their relatives should be warned against the hazards of self medicating with both prescribed and 'over the counter' drugs and the potential dangers when such medication is taken with alcohol. Such health promotion activities should be provided in appropriate settings, for example, social clubs used by the elderly, nursing homes and in pre-retirement classes.

Treatment and rehabilitation

For those elderly patients who require detoxification, treatment should be carried out within a hospital setting in view of the need for a high level of medical monitoring, and so as to treat any underlying physical and/or psychiatric complications. Elderly patients are more sensitive to relatively small doses of psychotropic medication due to the metabolic changes cited earlier and may require a longer period of detoxification. The use of drugs with a short half-life such as oxazepam or lorazepam is recommended to reduce the risk of confusion or delirium (Bienenfield, 1990). Similarly the use of disulfiram (antabuse) to help prevent relapse on alcohol should be used under close supervision and on a short-term basis since there is also a risk of precipitating a confusional state (Dunne, 1994).

Individual counselling and group therapy may be considered with some clients to address emotional difficulties such as bereavement and grief, loss of self-esteem and feelings of loneliness and alienation all of which might be antecedents to substance misuse. In addition, the involvement of a social worker to assist with any financial, legal and housing difficulties and to develop social networks with community agencies for the elderly will help to alleviate stress and isolation.

Summary of interventions

The interventions may be summarized:

- health advice given to clients, relatives and care givers regarding the risks associated with substance misuse;
- lengthier detoxification period using drugs with shorter half-lives e.g. oxazepam, lorazepam;
- individual counselling, group work and grief therapy;
- social work help with any financial, legal or housing problems;
- help to develop social networks.

CONCLUSION

Substance misuse represents a growing problem for a significant number of elderly people who are at a greater risk for medical and psychiatric complications. Thus far, heathcare professionals have been slow to respond. Pessimistic and fatalistic attitudes by clients, relatives and professionals as to the perceived benefits of interventions tend to militate against early identification and effective treatment outcomes. Addiction nurses have a crucial role to play in educating clients, their relatives and other professionals about the health problems associated with the misuse of substances and to help develop effective treatment strategies that are appropriate for this client group. Establishing close working links with hospital and community staff, general practitioners and residential care workers for the elderly will assist in the detection rate of elderly substance misusers.

REFERENCES

Atkinson, R.M. (1984) Substance use and abuse in late life, in *Alcohol and drug abuse in old age* (ed. R.M. Atkinson), American Psychiatric Press, Washington, DC, pp. 1–21.

Bienenfeld, D. (1990) Substance abuse in the elderly, in *Verwoerdt's clinical geropsychiatry*, 3rd edn (ed. D. Bienenfeld), Williams & Wilkins, Baltimore.

Bridgewater, R., Leigh, S., *et al.* (1987) Alcohol consumption and dependence in elderly patients in an urban community. *British Medical Journal*, **295**(6603), 884–5.

Bristow, M.F. and Clare, A.W. (1992) Prevalence and characteristics of at-risk drinkers among elderly acute medical in-patients. *British Journal of Addiction*, **87**(2), 291–94.

Caird, F.I. and Scott, P.J. (1986) *Drug-induced diseases in the elderly. Drug-induced disorders, Vol. 2*, Elsevier, Amsterdam.

Campbell, A.J. (1991) Drug treatment as a cause of falls in old age: a review of offending agents. *Drugs & Ageing*, **1**(14), 289–302.

Cooper, J.W. (1990) Drug-related problems in the elderly at all levels of care. *Journal of Geriatric Drug Therapy*, **4**, 79–83.

Cooper, J.W. (1994) Falls and fractures in nursing home patients receiving psychotropic drugs. *International Journal of Geriatric Psychiatry*, **9**, 975–80.

Dunne, F. (1994) Misuse of alcohol or drugs by elderly people. *British Medical Journal*, **308**(6829), 608–9.

Jones, D., Sweetnam, P.M., *et al.* (1980) Drug prescribing by GP's in England and Wales. Journal of Epidemiology and Community Health, **34**(2), 119–23.

Jones, D. (1992) Characteristics of elderly people taking psychotropic medication. *Drugs & Ageing*, **2**(5), 389–94.

Liberto, J.G., Oslin, D.W., *et al.* (1992) Alcoholism in older persons: A review of the literature. *Hospital and Community Psychiatry*, **43**(10), 975–84.

Malcolm, M.T. (1984) Alcohol and drug use in the elderly visited at home. *International Journal of addictions*, **19**(4), 411–18.

McInnes, E., Powell, J. (1994) Drug and alcohol referrals: are elderly substance abuse diagnoses and referrals being missed? *British Medical Journal*, **308**(6926), 444–46.

OPCS (Office of Population Censuses and Surveys) (1987) *Population projections, 1985–2041*, HMSO, London.

Saunders, P., Copeland, J., *et al.* (1991) Heavy drinking as a risk factor for depression and dementia in elderly men. *British Journal of Psychiatry*, **159**, 213–16.

Skegg, D. (1979) Prescribing for the elderly by British general practitioners, in *Drug treatment and prevention in cerebrovascular disorders* (ed. G. Tognori), Elsevier, North Holland BTO Medical Press, Holland.

Warren, J., Taylor, E., *et al.* (1985) Drug compliance in the elderly after discharge from hospital. *Pharmaceutical Journal*, **241**, 90–2.

Winnick, C. (1962) Maturing out of narcotic addiction. *Bulletin on Narcotics*, **14**(1), 1–7.

Wittington, F.J. (1983) Consequences of drug use, misuse and abuse, in *Drugs and the elderly* (eds M.D. Glantz, D.M. Peterson and F.J. Wittington), Research Monograph No. 32, NIDA, Rockville, MD.

Gay men, lesbians and substance misuse

13

G. Hussein Rassool

INTRODUCTION

During the past two decades there has been a growing awareness among clinicians and researchers that gay men and lesbians misuse drugs and alcohol in substantially greater proportions than the general population. Gay men, lesbians and bisexual men and women comprise a tangible minority population whose health-care needs are not usually met by mainstream health and substance misuse agencies. In addition, the issues of stigma, shame, homophobia and self-disclosure have compounded the problems of gay men and lesbians.

The advent of HIV and AIDS has exacerbated the whole process of caring and treating gay and lesbian substance misusers. It is acknowledged that HIV infection acquired through unprotected sexual intercourse can also be transmitted by contaminated injecting equipment, and gay men and lesbians with substance use problems may also acquire or transmit the infection through this route. From a public health perspective, it is important to determine the extent of injecting drug use among gay men and lesbian since injecting drug use is one of the primary sources of HIV transmission. The 'hidden' nature of this special population has made it difficult to obtain data and to estimate the incidence and prevalence rates of substance misuse among gay men and lesbians. Gay men and lesbians with substance use problems often need service provision specific to their needs. Addiction nurses and other healthcare professionals need to be more aware of the specific and diverse needs of this group and to gain more information about gender diversity to provide quality healthcare. In order to develop effective health education and health promotion activities, it became important to learn more about the nature and patterns of substance misuse among gay and bisexual men, and lesbians and their differing needs. Current research seems to establish that while alcohol and other drug misuse among gay men, lesbians and bisexuals are not dramatically different or worse than that of heterosexuals, different correlates and patterns exist and need to be understood in order to provide effective prevention and treatment (California Department of Alcohol and Drug Programs, 1992).

In this chapter, the nature and extent of substance misuse in gay men and lesbians will be presented and the problems and issues related to this special population will be examined. It will also address the addiction nurses' role in meeting the specific needs of these communities. Although the word community is used in this chapter when talking about gay men and lesbians, it is important to indicate that not all gay men or lesbians identify with a particular 'community'.

NATURE AND EXTENT OF SUBSTANCE MISUSE

Do gay men and lesbians people have more problems with alcohol and drugs than the heterosexual population? There is a dearth of literature available on the incidence and prevalence of substance misuse and addictive behaviour among gay men and lesbians in the UK. In the case of lesbians and bisexual women, much less is known about their use and misuse of alcohol and other psychoactive substances as compared to gay and bisexual men. Most of the studies related to the incidence and prevalence of drug and alcohol related problems among gay men and lesbians are from North American literature. Early research studies were mainly focused on estimating prevalence of alcohol among gay men, and it is only recently that this focus has shifted in studies relating to the use of illicit psychoactive substances (Morales and Graves, 1983; Stall and Wiley, 1988).

However, there is a growing notion that some gay men and lesbians misuse a wide range of psychoactive substances including alcohol, cannabis, amphetamines, cocaine, amyl nitrite and ecstasy. The Kelly study (1991) found that about 42% of gay and bisexual men reported using alcohol and or/drugs at 'problematic' levels. Alcohol was clearly the drug of choice for both men (75%) and women (66%); marijuana was the second most commonly used drug with 50% of the men and 38% of the women; and this was followed by the use of amyl nitrite (men (27%), women (3%)). In men, other psychoactive substances used were amphetamines, tranquillizers and cocaine (15%) and crack cocaine (7%). In women, painkillers, barbiturates and opiates were the third most frequently used drug, followed by amphetamines (9%) and crack cocaine (3%). Both groups of men and women were similar in their use of hallucinogens, barbiturates and heroin which range from 4% to 10%.

Recently, Bickelhaupt (1995) has provided a synopsis of seven research studies that examined the incidence of drug and alcohol addictions in gay and/or lesbian communities. Six of the studies were conducted in the USA and one in the Czech Republic. The findings show that between 20–35% of gay men and lesbian adults suffer from alcohol related problems, or use illicit, mind-altering drugs (Fifield, 1975; Kelly, 1991; Kus and Prochazka, 1991; Lohrenz et al., 1978;

Morales and Graves, 1983; Mosbacher, 1993; and Saghir and Robins, 1973). However, Bloomfield (1993) has argued that alcohol use among lesbians is no higher than heterosexuals and suggests that a similar study of homosexual men may reach the same result. Similarly, levels of alcohol use are said to be high among homosexual men, with drinking often leading to high-risk sexual behaviour (Friedman and Downey, 1994). This thesis has been refuted as there is little hard evidence available to substantiate this claim. In the UK, it is suggested that about one third to one fourth of gay men and lesbians misuse alcohol and other recreational psychoactive substances and it is estimated that lesbian women are particularly at risk of alcohol problems (Waterson, 1996).

However, some of the data available from the above studies are unreliable and based upon unrepresentative samples derived from the 'gay bar scene' who are more likely to have alcohol and drug problems. It has been suggested that research samples drawn from the gay bar scene may have inflated estimates of problem drinkers and problem drug users among gay men and lesbian (Friedman and Downey, 1994). Some of the studies focused on accessible but biased samples from institutions such as mental health centres and prisons. In addition, cross-cultural comparisons have not been made on the nature and pattern of substance misuse, especially illicit psychoactive substances. It is important to be cautious on extrapolating and generalizing from studies on the incidence of substance misuse in societies with different socioeconomic, political and healthcare systems.

Recognizing the methodological limitations and problems of earlier studies, more systematic and robust epidemiological surveys of substance misuse among gay men and lesbians have been advocated (Nardi, 1982). A three year prospective study, using a large randomized sample measuring the quantity and frequency of alcohol and drug misuse in gay men and heterosexual men, was undertaken by Stall and Wiley (1988). The results of the study indicated that 19% of gay men and 11% of heterosexual men (age 25–54) exhibited frequent/heavy drinking patterns (having 5 or more drinks on the same occasion). Statistically significant differences were found between gay men and heterosexual samples for those aged between 45–54 (13% and 7.6% respectively). Other findings showed that 82.9% of the gay men aged 25–34 had used marijuana/hashish in the past six months compared to 73.2% of the heterosexual sample. However, amyl nitrite (poppers) represented the largest significant difference in drug misuse in young gay men (58.8%) compared with 1.5% of the heterosexual sample using this drug. Another study by McKirnan and Peterson (1989a, 1989b) also found high prevalence of substance misuse in their sample of 3 400 gay men and lesbians. The results indicate that lesbian women and gay men were less likely than heterosexual women and men to abstain from alcohol and other psychoactive substances, and were more likely to be moderate users of these substances. An additional finding is that lifetime and past year use of marijuana and cocaine were found to be significantly higher among gay men and lesbian sample as compared to the general population.

The Research Symposium on Alcohol and Other Drug Problem Prevention Among Lesbians and Gay men (California Department of Alcohol and Drug

Programs, 1992) provides a summary of the significant differences between gay men, lesbians and the general population in the use of alcohol and other drugs. The findings are substantiated by scientifically rigorous research studies using large samples, in both urban and rural populations, in order to capture data from a more diverse population, The findings are summarized below:

- gay men appear to use alcohol in patterns similar to non-gay men;
- lesbians appear to use alcohol at higher rates than non-lesbian women;
- alcohol is the drug of choice for gay men and lesbians;
- gay men and lesbians use drugs at substantially higher rates than men and women in the general population;
- fewer gay men and lesbians abstain from alcohol than their general population counterparts;
- although more lesbians and gay men use alcohol than their general population counterparts, most appear to be moderate drinkers;
- as people get older their substance use tends to decrease. Among gay men and lesbians, this decrease is not as substantial as among the general population;
- although there is little evidence that addiction rates are higher among lesbians and gay men, some studies found that lesbians and gay men reported higher rates of substance use problems;
- there appears to be either 'more problem for the drink' among lesbians and gay men, or this population is more likely than the general population to admit problems related to substance misuse.

PROBLEMS AND ISSUES RELATED TO SUBSTANCE MISUSE

Gay men and lesbians face many problems because of the homophobia in our culture. According to Kominars (1995), 'homophobia is the irrational response to gay men and lesbians, or the idea of homosexuality. It is an irrational response, not a rational one. Whether gay men and lesbians "come out" or hide their sexual orientation or preference, most gay men and lesbians experience the effects of prejudice and stigmatization emanating from the homophobia of both society and healthcare professionals' (Irwin, 1992; Rose and Platzer, 1993).

There is evidence to suggest that an AIDS medical diagnosis and a history of injecting drug use were found to increase nurses' negative attitudes significantly towards patients and reduce their willingness to interact with these patients (Forrester and Murphy, 1992). The negative perceptions towards gay men and lesbians by healthcare professionals are also a barrier to help-seeking. Eliason (1993) stated that negative attitudes and misinformation can lead to poor quality of care and disrupt the nurse–patient relationships.

Furthermore, findings from alcohol treatment programmes suggest that many agencies do not address the sexual diversity and fail to address the specific needs of lesbians and gay men with alcohol-related problems (Gooch,1988). This unresponsiveness of service provision also applies to treatment programmes for those with drug-related problems. Weathers (1980) identified three major types of negative reaction that characterized this client group's experiences with alcohol agencies:

- refusal of services if the woman's lesbianism is known or suspected;
- provision of services on a limited basis, or with negative attitudes that are not conducive to support, growth, self-disclosure, or sobriety;
- provision of services directed toward isolating and 'curing' lesbianism as the primary problem, with little or no attention directed to alcohol-related problems.

Although these responses are a little out-of-date, in some way they still do reflect prevailing attitudes and perceptions towards gay men and lesbians. Despite the changes from service providers in their perception of gay men and lesbians, there is still a long way to go for this group to achieve parity with others within the healthcare system. Gay men and lesbians need resources specific to their needs and some of the issues that are unique to this population.

According to Kus and Smith (1995), gay men and lesbians have specific problems which may need attention in addition to the problems related to substance misuse. They identified several issues that include 'internalized homophobia' – 'seeing one's homosexuality as a negative rather than positive aspect of one's self'. The signs and symptoms of internalized homophobia, according to Kus (1995), include low self-esteem, chronic anxiety, inability to concentrate, treating gay men or lesbians poorly, passing as 'straight', physical illness, continual striving for high achievement and the inability to engage in same-sex sexual activity without the use of mind-altering psychoactive substances. However, both gay men and lesbians suffer from 'internalized homophobia', a state that is unique to this population. For gay and lesbian substance misusers, internalized homophobia will not disappear until sobriety is achieved and maintained through time (Kus, 1988). Many gay men and lesbians problem-drinkers do not recognize their internalized homophobia because it is being masked with alcohol and other mind-altering drugs (Kus and Smith, 1995).

According to Hetherington (1995) gay and lesbian couples are no exception in having problems related to issues such as public image, dieting, losing contact with own needs, goals and feelings, social isolation, boundary confusion and intimacy. Problems associated with the substance misuse include hepatitis, HIV infection, STD, and problems related to injecting drugs, such as septicaemia, thrombosis and abscess formation; and alcohol-related disorders. These problems are not in any way specific to lesbians and gay men but are also prevalent in heterosexual problem-drinkers and problem drug users.

In relation to gender difference, McKirnan and Peterson (1992) found that lesbians and gay men have different perceptions towards the co-existence between mental health problems and substance misuse. More lesbians than gay men stated that they drank or used drugs to cope with depression and anxiety, although the same number of lesbians and gay men reported mental health problems. It is argued that this finding illustrates how women's substance use has historically been perceived as a sign of mental illness, while gay men substance use is viewed as a physical illness (McKirnan and Peterson 1992).

Role of the addiction nurse

Addiction nurses need to have a greater awareness of the unique health needs of such clients, and examine their own cultural belief systems about sexuality. Nurses have a moral and professional responsibility to provide good, nonjudgemental care and there is no alternative 'opt-out' clause with this client group (UKCC, 1992; RCN, 1993). In meeting the healthcare needs of this population, addiction nurses must be familiar with the specific issues and problems associated with gay men and lesbians substance misusers. For instance, some gay men and lesbians may prefer self-help groups or specialized agencies related to their needs. A comprehensive assessment needs to be carried out in a nonjudgemental approach with the proviso of confidentiality.

Addiction nurses are well placed to provide specific care and harm-minimization educational activities related to safer sexual practices and safer drug use to this client group. Counselling and other intervention strategies should focus on areas of relationships, mental health problems, family issues, sexuality issues, leisure issues, legal issues and friendship networks. The involvement of partners is also of paramount importance in the care and treatment of those with substance misuse problems especially those who have been alienated from their families. The importance of meeting the spiritual needs of the gay community, and the spirituality in health and well-being of terminally ill gay men with HIV illness has been documented elsewhere (Kendall, 1994; Booth, 1995).

CONCLUSION

It is apparent that more research is needed into the incidence and prevalence of substance misuse and addictive behaviour in gay men and lesbians. Nursing research should focus on the health needs of gay men and lesbian substance misusers if we are to develop and implement specific treatment programmes effectively. The health issues relating to gay men and lesbians should also be examined in addiction nursing. It must be borne in mind that there are distinctive psychological, medical and social issues of HIV and gay men and lesbians. Different nursing and other health and social care interventions are required. There is a need to address gay men and lesbians health issues as part of the preparation and continuing education of addiction nurses and other healthcare professionals. Clear guidelines and policy changes in service provision are the necessary step in meeting the healthcare needs of this population.

Acknowledgement

I would like to thank Maeve Malley, Assistant Director of Newham Alcohol Advisory Service, London, for her comments and suggestions on this chapter.

REFERENCES

Bickelhaupt, E.E. (1995) Alcoholism and Drug Abuse in Gay and Lesbian Persons: A Review of Incidence Studies, in *Addiction and Recovery in Gay and Lesbians Persons* (ed. R.J. Kus), Haworth Press, Inc. New York.

Bloomfield, K (1993) A comparison of alcohol consumption between lesbians and heterosexual women in urban population. *Drug and Alcohol Dependence*, **33**(3), 257–69.

Booth, L. Fr. (1995) Spirituality and the Gay Community, in *Addiction and Recovery in Gay and Lesbians Persons* (ed. R.J. Kus), Haworth Press Inc., New York.

California Department of Alcohol and Drug Programs (1992) *Proceedings of the Research Symposium on Alcohol and Other Drug Problem Prevention Among Lesbians and Gay Men*, Sacramento, California.

Eliason, M.J. (1993) Cultural diversity in nursing care: the lesbian, gay, or bisexual client. *Journal of Transcultural Nursing*, **5**(1), 14–20.

Fifield, L. (1975) *On my way to nowhere: Alienated, isolated, drunk*, Los Angeles: Gay Community Services Center and Department of Health Services, County of Los Angeles.

Forrester, D.A. and Murphy, P.A. (1992) Nurses' attitudes toward patients with AIDS and AIDS-related risk factors. *Journal of Advanced Nursing*, **17**(10), 1260–66.

Friedman, R.C. and Downey, J.I. (1994) Homosexuality. *New England Journal of Medicine*, **331**(14), 923–30.

Gooch, S. (1988) Reapers after repression. *Nursing Standard*, **84**(29), 22–9.

Hetherington, C. (1995) Dysfunctional Relationship Patterns: Positive Changes for Gay and Lesbian People, in *Addiction and Recovery in Gay and Lesbians Persons* (ed. R.J. Kus), Haworth Press Inc., New York, pp. 41–55.

Irwin, R. (1992) Critical re-evaluation can overcome discrimination: providing equal standards of care for homosexual patients. *Professional Nurse*, **7**(7), 435–8.

Kelly, J. (ed) (1991) *San Francisco lesbian, gay and bisexual alcohol and other drugs needs assessment study: vol. 1*, EMT Associates Inc. Sacramento, CA.

Kendall, J. (1994) Wellness spirituality in homosexual men with HIV infection. *Journal of the Association of Nurses in Aids Care*, **5**(4), 28–34.

Kominars, S.B. (1995) Homophobia: The Heart of the Darkness, in *Addiction and Recovery in Gay and Lesbians Persons* (ed. R.J. Kus), Haworth Press Inc., New York, pp. 29–39.

Kus, R.J. (1988) Alcoholism and non-acceptance of gay self: The Critical link. *Journal of Homosexuality*, **15**(1–2), 25–41.

Kus, R.J. and Prochazka, I. (1991) *Alcoholism in gay Czechoslovak men: An incidence study*. Paper presented at the 36th International Institute on the Prevention and Treatment of Alcoholism, Stockholm, Sweden.

Kus, R.J. (ed) (1995) *Addiction and Recovery in Gay and Lesbians Persons*. Haworth Press Inc., New York.

Kus, R.J. and Smith, G.B. (1995) Referrals and Resources for Chemically Dependent Gay and Lesbian Clients, in *Addiction and Recovery in Gay and Lesbian Persons* (ed. R.J. Kus), Haworth Press Inc., New York, pp. 91–107.

Lohrenz, L., Connelly, J., Coyne, L. and Spase, K. (1978) Alcohol problems in several mid-western homosexual communities. *Journal of Studies on Alcohol*, **39**, 1959–63.

McKirnan, D. and Peterson, P. (1989a) Psychosocial and Cultural Factors in Alcohol and Drug Abuse: An Analysis of a Homosexual Community. *Addictive Behaviours*, **14**(5), 555–63.

McKirnan, D. and Peterson, P. (1989b) Alcohol and Drug Use among Homosexual Men and Women: Epidemiology and Population Characteristics. *Addictive Behaviours*, **14**(5), 545–53.

McKirnan, D. and Peterson, P. (1992) *Gay and Lesbian Alcohol Use: Epidemiological and Psychological Perspectives*. Paper presented at the Research Symposium on Alcohol and Other Drug Problem Prevention Among Lesbians and Gay Men, California Department of Alcohol and Drug Problems and EMT Group Inc., Los Angeles, August.

Morales, E.S. and Graves, M.A. (1983) *Substance abuse: Patterns and barriers to treatment of gay men and lesbians in San Francisco*, San Francisco Resources Center, San Francisco.

Mosbacher, D. (1993) Alcohol and other drug use in female medical students: A comparison of lesbians and heterosexuals. *Journal of Gay and Lesbians Psychotherapy*, **2**(1), 37–48.

Nardi, R. (1982) Alcoholism and Homosexuality: a theoretical perspective. *Journal of Homosexuality*, **7**(4), 9–25.

Rose, P. and Platzer, H. (1993) Confronting prejudice. *Nursing Times*, **49**(3), 52–4.

Royal College of Nursing (1993) *Refusal to Nurse: Guidance for Nurses*. RCN, London.

Saghir, M. and Robins, E. (1973) *Male and female homosexuality*, Williams and Wilkins, Baltimore.

Stall, R. and Wiley, J. (1988) A comparison of drug and alcohol use habits of heterosexual and homosexual men. *Drug and Alcohol Dependence*, **22**, 63–74.

United Kingdom Central Council (1992) *Professional Conduct for Nurses, Midwives and Health Visitors*, UKCC, London.

Waterson, J. (1996) Gender Divisions and drinking problems, in *Alcohol Problems in the Community* (ed. L. Harrison), Routledge, London.

Weathers, B. (1980) Alcoholism and the lesbian community, in *Alcoholism and Women* (eds M.C. Eddy and J. Ford), Kendall/Hunt, Dubunque, IA.

The use of psychoactive substances in young people

Mike Gafoor

14

INTRODUCTION

Substance misuse among young people is the source of much public concern and political debate. The inherent dangers associated with illicit drug use tend to evoke strong paternalistic responses from society concerning the need to protect the health and wellbeing of its future generations. Recent deaths associated with the drug ecstasy have generated widespread publicity and brought renewed calls for urgent government action. In its report 'Tackling Drugs Together' (1995) the government sets out as one of its aims 'to reduce the acceptability and availability of drugs to young people'. However, such claims are regarded by many healthcare workers to be unachievable in view of the government's liberal approach to legal drugs such as alcohol and tobacco. They argue that a failure to ban cigarette advertising and to increase the price of alcohol relative to other commodities can lead to an increase in the use of these substances particularly by young people (Plant and Plant, 1992). Also, it is a widely held view that the concerns expressed in relation to the dangers associated with illicit drugs are exaggerated in comparison to the large scale damage caused by excessive drinking and cigarette smoking.

Are the concerns over substance misuse among young people justified, or is it as Cohen (1972) describes it a 'moral panic due to the distorted mass media portrayal of the real and imagined excesses of young people'? Furthermore, it has been argued that the use of psychoactive substances by young people is a form of risk-taking behaviour which according to Irwin (1989) is 'a normal transitional behaviour during adolescence'. If this is so, what then should be the goal of prevention? Should it be to prevent the use of substances, their abuse, or the consequences of such abuse?

The purpose of this chapter is to examine briefly the nature and extent of substance use and misuse among young people and to identify the main risk factors associated with illicit drug use/misuse. It will also highlight the implications for prevention and treatment and how services could become more accessible and appropriate to the needs of this group.

NATURE AND EXTENT

Illicit drugs

The initiation and early stages of drug use typically occur during adolescence (Botvin and McAllsiter,1981) a period when young people experiment with a variety of behaviours and lifestyle patterns as part of the process of developing their own identity and independence. The use of illicit drugs such as cannabis, LSD, amphetamines and ecstasy is widely perceived as being part of a distinctive youth culture with shared social norms for fashion, music, and beliefs. However Plant and Plant (1992) suggest that, although illicit drug use among young people is now a common phenomenon, only a small percentage will do so regularly or will experience harmful consequences. In the UK most prevalence studies are based on self – reported illicit drug use rather than problem drug use in young people with rates between 5% (Brown and Lawton, 1988) and 20% (Swadi,1988). Cannabis remains the most commonly used illicit drug and, in his survey of 400 young people aged 16–24 years, Ford (1990) found that 42% had used cannabis, 13% amphetamines, 9% LSD, 5% cocaine and 2% heroin. Regarding problem drug use, Pritchard and colleagues (1986) in their study of 808 teenagers aged between 14–16, found 11% as drug abusers with 4% having serious problems.

Alcohol misuse

Most studies report around 90% of young people have at least tried a 'proper' drink by the age of 16 (Bagnall, 1988), and in a survey of drinking habits in England and Wales carried out by Goddard (1991) 10% males and 3% females (aged 18–24) had consumed more than 50 units per week respectively. Overall young people drink less than adults, but when they drink, they tend to drink in larger amounts (Harford and Grant,1987) and are therefore likely to suffer from acute effects such as blackouts, hangovers as well as aggressive behaviours. As in the case of illicit drug use, the drinking of alcohol by young people is associated with challenging parental and societal norms together with a desire to appear 'grown up'. For many, an increased availability of money and leisure time may encourage unsafe drinking habits. Problem drinking may also be linked with problem or deviant behaviour as the incidence of heavy drinking is higher among juvenile delinquents and young offenders (McMurran,1990).

RISK FACTORS AND PREVENTIVE INTERVENTIONS

Research evidence suggests that the use of substances among young people is the result of a complex interplay of social, personality, cognitive and behavioural factors (Jessor and Jessor, 1977). Social influences from the family, peer group and media may promote or facilitate the initiation of substance use (Botvin,1983). In addition psychological factors such as impulsiveness, rebelliousness, low assertiveness and low self esteem may tend to increase adolescents' susceptibility to such pressures. However, as already pointed out, use of substances does not necessarily lead to misuse and whether an adolescent substance user progresses to develop more severe problems with substance use depends upon a number of risk factors. These include early age of onset of substance use and/or conduct problems, co-existing severe conduct problems, poor academic performance, lower levels of parental attachment and a family history of substance abuse or dependence (Buckstein,1995). In other words, research data suggests that although substance use can occur in any individual, the risk of substance misuse is higher among those young people with the greater number of risk factors. Such risk factors also tend to correlate with other health related behaviours such as premature sexual activity and delinquency. According to Jessor (1982) 'one of the clearest facts to have emerged from the past decade of research is that there is substantial co-variation among many of these health-related behaviours, that is they tend to occur together within the same adolescent'. Thus, prevention strategies are more likely to be effective if they are targeted towards various high risk subgroups and address a wider range of dysfunctional behaviours and psychosocial problems. Table 14.1 provides a model for matching risk factors with prevention interventions.

Table 14.1 Matching risk factors with preventive interventions

Risk factors	Type of interventions
1 Individual	
• Peer influence	Skills-based interventions (education, social
• Poor social skills	skills training, changing attitudes and beliefs)
2 Personality	
• Conduct disorder	Referral to community mental health teams
• Anxiety/depression, stress-relief	Stress management
3 Family	
• Poor parental support/skills	Parent management training
• History of substance misuse	Family therapy
4 Social	
• Unemployment	Improve socioeconomic conditions
• Lack of recreational activities	Changes in policies/legislation
• Availability, price, social norms	Media campaigns

Case vignette

Jamie is 14 years old and comes from a middle-class background. He has been using solvents, mainly by sniffing cans of aerosols, since the age of 12, but the problem only recently came to light when he was found intoxicated at school. Jamie was referred to the school counsellor who contacted the community drug team and arranged for a joint assessment with the specialist nurse. James said that he sniffs on average around four cans of lighter fuel daily which he buys from several newsagents in order to conceal his problem. He liked the effects of solvents as it helped him to relax and take his mind off problems at home. He was concerned about his father's drinking which was a source of frequent arguments and fights at home.

Jamie was provided with information concerning the health risks of sniffing aerosols and advised against riding his bicycle while intoxicated. He was asked to keep a diary of the quantity and frequency, as well as relevant events which preceded his solvents use. He reluctantly agreed for his parents to attend subsequent appointments. Jamie's pattern of use was mainly centred around the lunch period at school, being on his own at home after school, and arguments with his parents. Both his parents acknowledged that the home situation had been difficult for Jamie but were unaware of their son's problem. It was then agreed for the specialist nurse to meet with Jamie for a few sessions during lunch time to help him to manage his cravings for solvents. He also met with the school counsellor to discuss his feelings regarding his parents' marital difficulties. His mother was able to come home earlier from work and accompanied Jamie to swimming classes at the local pool. His father managed to reduce his alcohol consumption and later took up the offer of attending a marriage guidance clinic with his wife. Jamie has now been solvent free for six months.

Nursing interventions

Assessment

The purpose of the assessment of a young substance misuser is to identify the nature and extent of substance misuse, along with the degree of physical and psychosocial dysfunction in order to make the most appropriate treatment interventions. Most young substance misusers rarely self refer for treatment and may be referred by their parents, GPs, social workers, school nurses or community workers. It is necessary, therefore, for the specialist nurse to engage the young client by conducting the assessment interview in a sensitive and non-judgmental manner and to provide reassurances regarding confidentiality.

An awareness of the risk factors mentioned above together with information regarding patterns of use, negative consequences, context of use and control of use should enable the addiction nurse to determine the severity of the problem. Urine testing for drug screening and collateral information from parents and other relevant sources will also aid the assessment process.

Special needs and implications for treatment

Substance misuse treatment services in the UK have been traditionally geared towards meeting the needs of individuals in their 20s and 30s, and more severely dependent substance misusers. Such services have been regarded as inappropriate in meeting the needs of younger substance misusers who differ from other clients in that their history of substance misuse is shorter, they rarely manifest long-term side-effects of substance misuse, and they are more vulnerable to peer pressure to use drugs and alcohol. Furthermore, their cognitive development is not fully complete and they face difficulties in internalizing and implementing treatment concepts. It is not surprising that 50% of adolescents drop out of treatment (Longabaugh, 1987).

Young substance misusers are not attracted by long-term treatment goals such as preventing liver cirrhosis from alcohol misuse or lung cancer from cigarette smoking (Botvin et al., 1984). Immediate and short-term goals need to be designed in order to increase motivation to treatment. The aim is to provide an accessible and flexible treatment setting that can respond to their unique needs and may require greater involvement from GPs and other members of the primary healthcare teams. These needs may include treatment of dependence, but are also likely to include addressing social or psychological difficulties or health problems.

Health education programmes should be an integral part of any substance misuse treatment programme as well as providing opportunities for the teaching of parenthood skills to the parents of young substance misusers. Most adolescents are still in school and live at home and need a great deal of family involvement in their treatment.

CONCLUSION

The use of psychoactive substances is common among young people and the development of substance misuse appears related to social and personality factors as well as family history of substance misuse and early age of onset of substance use. Because young people are not fully developed in their social, cognitive and emotional functioning, they require specific treatment and intervention strategies that take into account their developmental needs. Addiction nurses as specialist clinicians have an important role in the assessment, prevention and treatment of substance misuse among this section of the population.

REFERENCES

Bagnall, G. (1988) Use of alcohol, tobacco and illicit drugs amongst 13 year-olds in three areas of Britain. *Drug and Alcohol Dependence*, **22**(23), 241–51.

Botvin, G.J. and McAllister, A. (1981) Cigarette smoking among children and adolescents: Causes and prevention, in *Annual Review of Disease Prevention* (ed. C.B. Arnold), Springer, New York.

Botvin, G.J. (1983) Prevention of Adolescent Substance Abuse Through the Development of Personal and Social Competence, in: *Preventing Adolescent Drug Abuse: Intervention Strategies*, NIDA Research Monograph, **47**, 115–40.

Botvin, G.J., Barker, E., Renick, N.L. *et al.* (1984) A cognitive behavioural approach to substance abuse prevention. *Journal of Addictive Behaviour*, **9**(2), 137–47.

Brown, C. and Lawton, J. (1988) *Illicit Drug Use in Portsmouth and Havant*, Policy Studies Institute, London.

Buckstein, O.G. (1995) Development, Risk and Consequences, in *Adolescent Substance Abuse: Assessment, Prevention, and Treatment*, (ed. O.G. Buckstein), Wiley-Interscience, New York, pp. 53–72.

Cohen, S. (1972) *Folk Devils and Moral Panic*, Granada, London.

Ford, N. (1990) *Psychoactive Drug Use, Sexual Activity and Aids awareness of young people in Bristol*, Institute of Population Studies, University of Exeter..

Goddard, E. (1991) *Drinking in England and Wales in the late 1980s*. HMSO, London.

Harford, T.C. and Grant, B. (1987) Psychosocial factors in adolescent drinking contexts. *Journal of Studies on Alcohol*, **48**(6), 551–57.

Irwin, C.E. (1989) Risk-taking behaviours in the adolescent patient: are they impulsive? *Paediatric Annals*, **18**(2), 122–30.

Jessor, R. and Jessor, S.L. (1977) *Problem Behaviour and Psychosocial Development: A Longitudinal Study of Youth*. Academic Press, New York.

Jessor, R. (1982) Critical issues in research on adolescent health promotion, in *Promoting Adolescent Health: A Dialogue on Research and Practice* (eds T. Coates, A. Petersen, A. and C. Perry), Academic Press, New York.

Longabaugh, R. (1987) Longitudinal outcome studies, in *Alcoholism: Origins and Outcome* (eds R.M. Rose and J. Barrett), Raven Press, New York.

McMurran, M. (1990) Young offenders and alcohol, in *Applying Psychology to Young Offenders* (ed. M. McMurran), British Psychological Society, Leicester, pp. 45–9.

Plant, M. and Plant, M. (1992) Illicit Drug Use, in *Risk-Takers: Alcohol, Drugs, Sex and Youth* (eds M. Plant and M. Plant), Tavistock/Routledge, London, pp. 40–8.

Pritchard, C., Fielding, M., *et al.* (1986) Incidence of drug and solvent abuse in 'normal' fourth and fifth year comprehensive school children – some socio-behavioural characteristics. *British Journal of Social Work*, **16**, 341–51.

Swadi, H. (1988) Drug and substance use among 3,333 London adolescents. British Journal of Addiction, **83**(8), 935–42.

Tackling Drugs Together (1995), HMSO, London.

15

Homelessness and addictions

Mike Gafoor

INTRODUCTION

In the UK, the homeless population has doubled in recent years (Department of the Environment, 1990) and, although there is uncertainty among professionals as to what constitutes homelessness, it has been suggested that 1–2 million people may be homeless (Scott, 1993). The problem is often associated with people sleeping rough and this visible subgroup attracts considerable media and public attention especially during the winter months when their problems are more apparent. In fact this group represents only a small proportion of the homeless population, the majority of whom have access to some form of accommodation such as hostels, shelters and bed and breakfast lodgings (Black *et al.*, 1991).

Scott (1993) argues that homelessness should not merely relate to the issue of housing but to 'anyone who lacks adequate shelter, resources and community ties'. Such a definition is more appropriate because it also takes into account the social marginalization experienced by homeless people and assists in the development of methods to meet their complex needs. Controversy also exists as to the causes of homelessness and whether it is fundamentally a health or an economic problem (Rossi *et al.*,1987). Factors such as unemployment, poverty, family problems, eviction, substance misuse and mental illness have all been cited as both causes and consequences of homelessness. What is without doubt, however, is that the prevalence of substance misuse, physical and psychiatric morbidity is higher among homeless people than among the domiciled population.

The aims of this chapter are to identify the main difficulties experienced by the homeless substance misuser and to examine the important contribution of addiction nurses in responding to their needs.

NATURE AND EXTENT

The stereotypical image of a homeless substance misuser is the vagrant alcoholic who snarls at passers by or the emaciated street beggar with a dog. It is clear, however, that homeless substance misusers are not an homogenous group and include single men, women, families and mentally ill people. Recent studies have shown a high prevalence of substance misuse among homeless people with rates between 25–75% (Shanks *et al.*, 1994; Newton *et al.*, 1994). Alcohol misuse appears to be a more common problem and is estimated to be 6–7 times higher among homeless men and 15–30 times higher in homeless women than in the general population (Fischer and Breakey,1992). Furthermore, substance misuse co-exists with mental illness in 20% of homeless people and a third have a major affective disorder. High levels of criminal activity particularly relating to intoxication are also another feature of homelessness (Lamb, 1984).

In addition to their social and psychological problems, homeless substance misusers suffer from a high incidence of physical problems and have a mortality rate that is three times more than people without a home. Studies show that there is a positive relationship between the duration of homelessness and physical morbidity. Chest infections such as bronchitis and tuberculosis are particularly common as well as peripheral vascular disease, peptic ulcers and traumatic injuries. Recently, Klee and Morris (1995) have suggested that homeless drug users are more likely to be involved in HIV risk-taking behaviour through increased sharing of injecting equipment and casual, unprotected sex.

ACCESS TO HEALTH CARE

Despite high levels of physical, social and psychological morbidity, the utilization of healthcare services by homeless people remains low and most are not registered with a GP (Scott and Boustead, 1991). While it is possible that many GPs are reluctant to add this unpopular group of clients to their lists, an alternative explanation might be that the homeless do not perceive healthcare as a priority over more pressing needs such as food, clothing and shelter. Because of their transient lifestyle and nature of their problems, many homeless substance misusers find it difficult to keep hospital appointments or to comply with institutional bureaucratic rules. As a result they are less likely to be referred to specialist services, and even when they do attend many fail to complete treatment (Finn, 1985). It has also been suggested that the new NHS reforms tend to exclude homeless people from healthcare as many district health authorities responsible for purchasing healthcare services for the resident population have 'disowned' the homeless as residents (Black *et al.*, 1991)

Role of the nurse

Nurses can play an important role in responding to the diverse needs of the homeless substance misuser. As already mentioned, such clients are difficult to access in view of their social disaffiliation and reluctance to engage in traditional treatment programmes. Forging links with agencies for the homeless and helping staff both to recognize and manage clients with drug and alcohol problems would ensure that care is provided in a setting most suited to their needs. Health education regarding the effects of drugs and alcohol on physical, social and mental health should be provided as well as strategies for reducing the use of such substances. In cases where admission to hospital is required for detoxification and/or treatment of physical and psychiatric complications, the nurse can facilitate this process by liaising with specialist services on behalf of the client. In addition to their healthcare needs, the homeless substance misuser requires social support in areas such as housing, financial benefits and employment and the nurse can play a significant role in helping clients to access social and welfare agencies.

Case vignette

Fred is 48 years old and has a history of alcohol misuse that dates back to his early 20s. Over the years his drinking has had a devastating effect on his life with two failed marriages, loss of jobs and numerous convictions for drunk-related offences. He had also been hospitalized on several occasions after being injured fighting or falling over while intoxicated. Fred is well known at the local night-shelter and has been a regular client there since he was evicted by his landlady for starting a fire in his bedsit two years ago. His previous admissions to hospital for alcohol detoxification were usually precipitated by concerns over his physical and mental state. It has never been possible for Fred to remain in hospital long enough to find him stable accommodation. On leaving hospital, he would quickly return to the street drinking subculture and begging for money from passers by.

At the next assessment meeting with Fred, the addiction nurse invited the social worker responsible for funding residential services for substance misusers and the healthcare worker of a 'dry' hostel for homeless drinkers to attend. It was arranged for Fred to be detoxified at the hostel, with the addiction nurse visiting regularly to monitor his care and to support the hostel staff during the detoxification process. This was completed successfully and Fred remained at the hostel for a further six months before moving into permanent accommodation. He was helped to find work as a part-time gardener with the local church and attends Alcoholic Anonymous meetings regularly.

CONCLUSION

Homeless people represent one of the most disenfranchized groups in our society and present with multiple needs relating to their physical and mental state and substance misuse. Because of their social isolation (detachment) and transient lifestyles, their healthcare needs cannot be adequately met in traditional healthcare settings. Policy planners and healthcare workers need to be more imaginative and innovative in order to access this group. The setting up of satellite health clinics and the use of community health workers would encourage greater utilization of health services by this group as well as ensuring that clients are seen in appropriate settings. Many homeless individuals have difficulties in gaining access to primary care as many GPs are reluctant to take such clients on to their lists. Nurses have an important advocacy role in helping clients to register with a GP and in co-ordinating their care between psychiatric, substance misuse and primary care agencies. Homeless people are a microcosm of our society: being homeless should not equate with being healthless.

REFERENCES

Black, M.E. and Scheuer, M.A. (1991) Utilisation by homeless people of acute hospital services in London. *British Medical Journal*, **303**(6808), 958–61.

Department of the Environment (1990) *Action of Local Authorities in Discharging Duties under the 1985 Housing Act,* HMSO, London.

Finn, P. (1985) Decriminalization of public drunkenness: response of the healthcare system. *Journal of Studies on Alcohol*, **46**(1), 7–23.

Fischer, P.J. and Breakey, W.R. (1992) The epidemiology of alcohol, drug and mental disorder among homeless persons. *American Psychologist*, **46**(1), 1115–28.

Klee, K. and Morris, J. (1995) Factors that characterize street injectors. *Addiction*, **90**(6), 837–41.

Lamb, R. (1984) Deinstitutionalization and the homeless mentally ill, in *The Homeless Mentally ill* (ed. R. Lamb), American Psychiatric Association, Washington DC.

Newton, J.R. and Geddes, J.R. (1994) Mental health problems of the Edinburgh 'roofless'. *British Journal of Psychiatry*, **165**(4), 537–40.

Rossi, P., Wright, J., *et al.* (1987) The urban homeless: estimating composition and size. *Science*, **235**(4794), 1336–41.

Scott, J. and Boustead, M. (1991) Characteristics of homeless adults in temporary accommodation. *British Journal of Clinical and Social Psychiatry* (Suppl. on Poverty), **7**, 182–87.

Scott, J. (1993) Homelessness and mental illness. *British Journal of Psychiatry*, **162**, 314–24.

Shanks, N.J., George, S.L., *et al.* (1994) Who are the homeless? *Public Health*, **108**(1), 11–9.

Offenders and addiction nursing

16

Bridget Kilpatrick and Jim Carroll

INTRODUCTION

There has been a long relationship between substance misuse and offending and illegal behaviour. Yet the intricacies of the relationship are not always clear cut or apparent. We are accustomed to hearing about alcohol and its role in contributing to offences of drink-driving, theft, criminal damage and violence but when crimes involve the use of other drugs the relationship is not quite so evident. There are burglaries, shoplifting offences and thefts committed to provide funds to maintain opiod and crack cocaine use. Individuals may also become involved in prostitution or fraud offences. Non-sexual crimes of violence may be committed under the effects of stimulant drugs or a combination of sedative drugs taken. Questioning about an alleged offence committed may not reveal a significant dependence upon a controlled drug since the misusers may well feel reluctant to add to their problems by admitting to substance misuse.

Staff working in substance misuse services are used to asking their clients about offending behaviour when undertaking an assessment, and have often provided court reports for clients answering charges. It is common for staff to feel that clients were only approaching them for a favourable court report and that they had no sincere interest in changing their substance misuse habits. The extent and nature of drug misuse, the advent of harm reduction principles and endorsement of non-custodial sentencing alternatives have led to services seeing misusers at different stages in their substance misuse career. Hence, services have adjusted pragmatically and are less likely to adhere to a belief that clients can only be seen if they approach a service voluntarily and seek only abstinence.

This chapter describes some of the criminal justice settings in which substance misusers may be found and makes suggestions about strategies that can be considered in response by addiction nurses working either directly in criminal justice agencies or in conjunction with them.

PARTNERSHIPS WITH CRIMINAL JUSTICE AGENCIES

Nurses working in designated addiction services have been affected by changes in the criminal justice system. In services such as smaller community teams it would not be unusual for pre-sentence reports to have been supplied by a nurse, as key worker. Also, for the nurse to have been involved in collaborative ventures with probation services (though not in Scotland which does not have a separate proba- tion service) for example contributions to community courses for offenders, under- taking pre-release prison visits with the probation officer, offering assessments and counselling to prisoners released early and working within prisons to offer health education. Currently, both collaborative ventures and multiagency co-operation between criminal justice and drug services are recommended in the recent gov- ernment strategy document to address the drugs problem for England (Tackling Drugs Together, 1995) and by the Criminal Justice Working Group (ACMD, 1991, 1994). Such developments involve diverse organizations including the health ser- vice, social services, police, probation service and prisons.

Any working partnerships require considerable preparatory planning to take into account whether different organizational philosophies, traditions and practices may be reconciled to promote inter-agency co-operation so as to stand above iso- lated, collaborative examples built upon individual energies and local relation- ships. Effective liaison between the probation service and drug treatment agencies has been the theme of recent work by the Advisory Council on the Misuse of Drugs. The Criminal Justice Working Group has been concerned to establish effective partnerships (ACMD, 1991). Nurses have been recruited by drug treat- ment services to undertake work with offenders in conjunction with probation ser- vices. However, it is felt that this partnership has not settled into a useful collaborative venture and that tensions remain which are likely to slow the pace of reform in England and Wales (Dorn and Lee, 1995). However, in Scotland the links between the drug and alcohol agencies and the law courts are reported as offering more success (Baldwin and Mc Millan, 1993).

Many substance misusers end up in prisons where there is concern not only about those who remain involved in drug-taking but also about the HIV risk-taking behaviour of sharing injecting equipment in institutional settings. Nurses who have worked in prisons as healthcare providers have had to get to grips with the real problems posed by substance misuse in an inmate population (Burrows, 1994; 1995). Criticisms over the quality of healthcare in prisons have been made in order to raise the standard of care so that it is compatible to community health service provision. The nursing service for prisoners has sought to increase the number of registered nurses working in prisons so as to offer an eclectic response to the phys- ical and psychological health problems of the inmates (Willmott, 1994).

Education and training in substance misuse is seen as crucial. The policy and strategy document of the prison healthcare service on drug misuse involves all healthcare staff in the identification and throughcare of drug misusers. This extends to the assessment, provision of an individual treatment plan, monitoring, establishment of liaison system with appropriate outside agencies and making provision for continued care and treatment upon release into the community (HM Prison Service, 1995). Nurses working within the prison healthcare system and those outside drug services are well placed to create and maintain links in order to improve treatment outcomes.

Addiction and Offending

The definition of a drug misusing offender is someone who, either offends:

- directly as a result of their misuse of controlled drugs; or
- because their misuse of controlled drugs has caused or contributed to their offences (ACMD, 1991).

This definition is specifically related to drugs but it is possible to retain it, when considering alcohol. Public order offences are usually related to alcohol misuse while acquisitive crimes, such as theft, are usually committed to provide funds to continue drinking or drug taking. Not all offenders would agree that they have a substance misuse problem and not all substance misusers offend, though there are undoubtedly links between offending and addictive behaviours. Offending and related substance misuse need not imply an offender is alcohol or drug dependent as offending may be linked with non-dependent misuse of a substance.

The task is to identify the exact nature of the relationship and to offer an appropriate intervention that is understood by the client. The opportunity to tease out and discuss a client's routine substance use is not as obvious to a nurse who is used to working in a designated addiction service with clients. There may be reluctance to disclose the nature and extent of substance misuse as admission may be felt to compound an already difficult forensic situation. It may fracture a sense of an individual's ability to function psychologically and the substance misuse may not be known to the offender's close friends or family.

Criminal justice settings

Substance misusers may be found at various settings within the criminal justice system and intervention by a nurse attached to a substance misuse service may be considered at many stages once a charge has been formally made. (A visit made before this stage by a forensic medical examiner can offer an opportunity to provide advice, information and treatment about the arrested person's substance misuse, but this is a medical and not a nursing role.)

Developments in criminal justice settings involving addiction services and nurses have been patchy, formed in an *ad hoc* manner and may not endure the passage of experience, time and evaluation. A conference by the Regional Drug and Alcohol Team, St George's Hospital, explored some of the initiatives in operation, and found varying levels of achievement. For example, a willingness by the police to arrange contact with a substance misuse service, after a formal caution or warning has been issued, may be tempered by difficulties in trying to develop links between police and drug services, in arranging access and establishing boundaries to the scheme (Annual Consultative Day, Drugs and Crime, 1995).

Magistrate courts process many drinking and drug-taking offenders and provide opportunities for court-based substance misuse intervention. A study of three court based-intervention schemes for alcohol related public-order offences among 17 to 24 year-olds revealed that there was a good response in the court setting to brief intervention techniques of a screening interview, supplemented by self-help manuals and the option of further assessment and education where required (Baldwin and McMillan, 1993). Outreach and diversionary schemes (interventions with offenders referred to addiction services) at courts may be perceived as demanding upon time, staff experience and resources for smaller addiction services. However, they offer clients, who might not ordinarily present at addiction services, further opportunities for offending and addictive behaviours to be explored in a group. Practical problems such as some offenders being of no fixed abode, negotiation with other catchment area addiction services, following-up clients, selection of appropriate interventions and the establishment of effective interdisciplinary relationships require strategic planning if they are to develop and become a local resource.

Bail schemes and bail hostels are a further opportunity to help substance misusers who are otherwise likely to be remanded in custody. There is a perceived under utilization of bail schemes for substance misusers but addiction nurses should develop links with hostels in their catchment area and initiate healthcare interventions. After conviction, substance misusers may receive a community sentence such as a probation order. Attached to the order may be a requirement for the offender to receive treatment for alcohol or drug dependency. An addiction nurse may be involved in this sentencing option, undertaking joint work with the offender and the probation service.

NATURE AND EXTENT OF SUBSTANCE MISUSE IN PRISON

Prisons cover a range of features: high security to open establishments; remand services; sentences ranging from short, medium to long; and adult or young offender institutions. Across the range of prison establishments there are perceived high levels of injecting drug use and of unprotected anal intercourse between men. There is also the potential for transmitting infections such as hepatitis B and HIV, and this has heightened concerns over the level and pattern of drug misuse and sexual behaviour in prisons. There is no doubt that substance misuse has been found among sentenced prisoners. Prevalence rates of substance misuse were found to be 12% in adult male and young offender prisoners (Gunn *et al.*, 1991; Maden *et al.*, 1991). Surveys about the drug use of sentenced prisoners in England and Wales in the six months prior to imprisonment found rates of drug dependence to be 11% in males and 23% in females (Gunn, 1991).

In Scotland, 32% of male drug users were injecting regularly before imprisonment (Shewan *et al.*, 1994a) and 28% had injected drugs before imprisonment in a male and female sample (Power *et al.*, 1994). Not all injectors in the community continue injecting when imprisoned and rates of injecting drugs use during imprisonment dropped to 11% (Shewan *et al.*, 1994a) and 8% (Power *et al.*, 1994). The injectors who continued, and those not able to continue with the oral substitute drugs prescribed before custody (Shewan *et al.*, 1994b), are thus more likely to use shared injecting equipment.

There is no one uniform group of substance misusers in prison; not all will require treatment on admission, some may benefit from healthcare within the prison, others may require further assessment and treatment not available within prison. In a purposive sample in four Scottish male adult prisons, prisoners were categorized under a number of headings: non-user of any drugs; alcohol users only; poly-users and non-injectors; ex-injectors; current injectors in the community but not continuing to inject in prison; current injectors in the community; injectors during previous imprisonment, and injectors during current sentence (Shewan *et al.*, 1994c). While many of the injectors will have been using, mainly or solely, opiods others may have been benzodiazepine and stimulant injectors, the latter group not frequently in contact with mainstream addiction services.

Healthcare provision

Contact with healthcare services for inmates may be complemented by staff from outside substance misuse services coming into prisons to work or collaborate on pre- and early-release schemes. There are however unique features associated with working in prisons. Nurses employed by prisons are both clinicians and custodians. Thus, a tension exists to maintain the balance of both their traditional caring role, which has to survive, along with the habitual custodial duty of the prison. Nurses have to adjust to working in a prison environment and have felt they were popular with other staff (Burrows, 1995). Issues such as prison policy on the permitted provision of cleaning agents (for injecting equipment) and the denied availability of condoms have attracted divergent responses (Payne, 1995). The recruitment of nurses into a private sector profit-making prison (McMillan, 1994) adds to these ethical considerations.

Healthcare interventions

Essentially the role of intervention with substance misuse offenders in the criminal justice system should be no different from those who are not involved, particularly if the aim of prison healthcare is to offer a service equitable to the health service outside. The impact of HIV/AIDS has led to the establishment of inter-mediate goals frequently referred to as the harm-reduction principles. These involve more flexible prescribing and less emphasis on total abstinence as an immediate goal. In institutional settings however, abstinence rather than mainte-nance remains the option for drug misusers.

Prisons have many health problems to contend with, arising out of a population with a rate of psychiatric disorder at 37% (Gunn *et al.*, 1991), 46% having med-ical problems upon arrival and a higher than national average of reporting sick (Burrows, 1995). However, the criminal justice system expects nurses to deal effectively with many offenders with various problems arising out of substance misuse. The needs of offenders who have ceased substance misuse should not be ignored as this could lead to relapse both in the prison and upon discharge. Offenders will have their own views on their links with substance misuse, and the views of a professional may not be so evident to the individual prisoner. Until the links made by the professional are accepted, it is unlikely that offenders will change their behaviour pattern.

There are undoubtedly constraints within the prison system for effective inter-vention to be implemented for incarcerated substance misusers. There is concern that compulsory urine testing for detection of drugs will make drug misusers switch from drugs with a longer half-life such as cannabis and benzodiazepines, to those with a relatively short half-life, such as heroin which is arguably more harmful. The likely impact of compulsory testing therefore could be detrimental and construed as yet another punishment rather than aiding rehabilitation. Interventions aimed at reducing the level of drug misuse in prisons are officially enshrined in government strategy and nurses are one of several disciplines in pris-ons who develop a range of initiatives embracing health advice and information, education, counselling and treatment.

The idea that prisoners should be able to serve their sentences in prisons close to their home community should enable local substance misuse services and other allied agencies to establish and retain links. It is debatable, however, whether this actually occurs – prisons are still perceived as difficult places for outside services to gain access and undertake therapeutic work, although the position has certainly improved with collaboration welcomed by prisoners, prisons and outside services. To effect changes in working practices can take time and invoke anxiety among staff as they get to grips with the many individual and institutional problems caused by substance misuse. These include the pressure placed upon prisoners and visitors to supply drugs, debts over drug deals, infection risks from shared inject-ing equipment, continued risk-taking behaviour, overdoses and other forms of self-harm (Burrows, 1994).

The range of direct and indirect problems associated with substance misuse involve physical and psychological health considerations as well as problems associated with education, work skills, housing and relationship difficulties, all of which occur in a setting isolated from family and peer support. Collaboration with outside agencies to undertake specific aspects of a substance misuse rehabilitation programme and to liaise with rehabilitative agencies at the pre-release stage are vital to reach certain offenders who have little or no previous contact with services. A failure to intervene is not contradictory to criminal justice aims, even though it is not always clear whether offender-rehabilitation rather than offender-punishment is the guiding principle of custody.

Substance misuse rehabilitation schemes do exist, such as a methadone reduction programme in Winchester, Hampshire but these may be subject to local arrangements. The establishment of drug-free areas, voluntary urine testing and programme participation by volunteer prisoners at Downview prison, Surrey, with rehabilitation and education provided by both prison and outside agencies is one example. In one prison, a drug reduction programme has been introduced to support newly arrived prisoners experiencing drug withdrawal from opioids and benzodiazepines; to provide information on drug-related harm, to offer an opportunity to address a drug-free lifestyle, to facilitate behaviour change and to reduce or stabilize drug use. Both prisoners and prison management advocated reduction prescribing rather than maintenance prescribing, but the Scottish Prison Service indicated that maintenance prescribing is acceptable for short-term or remand sentences only (Shewan *et al.* 1994d).

Care plans need to be individually tailored to the individual offender and require the co-operation and active participation of the offender to identify their needs and the establishment of, at least, short-term goals. Treatment methods include reduction prescribing, education, physical fitness training, social skills training, stress management training, improvement of self-concept, coping and relapse prevention skills (Burrows, 1994). Both individual and group counselling can be offered by a multi-disciplinary team of prison staff and outside services employed to deliver the interventions.

CONCLUSION

The criminal justice agencies and substance misuse services working together at first seem to involve the two irreconcilable aims of punishment and rehabilitation. To recognize a distinction between these aims is necessary but, if we are to meet the needs of people who both display offending and addictive behaviour, then we must develop a practice which resolves these differences. It is hoped that addiction services have shifted from the position of being unwilling to see an ambivalent client because of the presence of a pending court case. Likewise services have to be prepared to offer both less motivated and more motivated substance misusers help at various stages through the criminal justice process and this help need not cease once a client is arrested or imprisoned. Nurses are well represented in outside addiction services and developments in the nursing care of prisoners offer prospects to undertake work with substance misusers in prisons. The opening up of prisons to outside addiction services, to undertake information and education further breaks down existing barriers, real or imagined, and will help to remove the past separation of outside from prison healthcare. As many substance misusers remain hidden to outside services and seldom seek help without some element of coercion being present, it is not surprising that the identification and management of substance misuse is made easier in prisons.

The criminal justice system is a wide one, with many participating agencies represented between police arrest and release from imprisonment. Initiatives to provide healthcare to individuals with addiction and offending behaviour are a challenge as further needs of such people are addressed.

REFERENCES

Advisory Council on the Misuse of Drugs (1991) *Drug misusers and the criminal justice system, Part I: community resources and the probation service*, HMSO, London.

Advisory Council on the Misuse of Drugs (1994) *Drug misusers and the criminal justice system, Part II: police, drug misusers and the community*, HMSO, London.

Annual Consultative Day, Drugs and Crime, 8 December 1995, Regional Drug and Alcohol Team, St George's Hospital, London.

Baldwin, S. and McMillan, J. (1993) Down to zero: feasibility study of court-based brief interventions with drinking offenders in England and Wales. *Addiction Research*, **1**(2), 157–68.

Burrows, R. (1994) Fighting addiction in prisons. *Nursing Times*, **90**(24), 30–2, June 15–21.

Burrows, R. (1995) Captive care: changes in prison nursing. *Nursing Standard*, **10**(22), 29–31, Feb. 22–28.

Dorn, N. and Lee, M. (1995) Mapping probation practice with drug using offenders. *The Howard Journal*, **34**(4), 314–25.

Gunn, J., Maden, A. and Swinton, M. (1991) Treatment needs of prisoners with psychiatric disorders. *British Medical Journal*, **303**(6798), 338–41.

HM Prison Service (1995) *Drug Misuse in prison: Policy and Strategy*, HMSO, London.

Maden, A., Swinton, M. and Gunn, J. (1990) Women in prison and use of illicit drugs. *British Medical Journal*, **301**(6761), 1133.

Maden, A., Gunn, J., and Swinton, M. (1991) Drug dependence in prisoners. *British Medical Journal*, **302**(6781), 880.

McMillan, I. (1994) Healthy inside. *Nursing Times*, **90**(40), 14–5.

Payne, D. (1995) Protection package. *Nursing Times*, **91**(30), 20–1.

Power, K.G., Markova, I., Rowlands, A., McKee, K.J. and Kilfedder, C. (1994) Inmates self-perceived risk of HIV infection inside and outside Scottish prisons. *Health Education Research*, **9**(1), 47–55.

Shewan, D., Gemmell, M. and Davies, J.B. (1994a) Behavioural change amongst drug injectors in Scottish prisons. *Social Science and Medicine*, **39**(11), 1585–6.

Shewan, D., Gemmell, M. and Davies, J.B. (1994b) *Drug use and prison*, occasional paper no. 5, Scottish Prison Service, Edinburgh.

Shewan, D., Gemmell, M. and Davies, J.B. (1994c) *Drug use and Scottish prisons*, occasional paper no. 6, Scottish Prison Service, Edinburgh.

Shewan, D., McPherson, S., Reid, M.M. and Davies, J.B. (1994d) *Evaluation of the Saughton drug reduction programme*, occasional paper no. 11, Scottish Prison Service, Edinburgh.

Tackling Drugs Together (1995). A strategy for England 1995–1998, Cm 2846, HMSO, London.

Willmott, Y. (1994) Career opportunities in the nursing service for prisoners. *Nursing Times*, **90**(24), 29–30.

17

Substance misuse and mental health

Mike Gafoor

INTRODUCTION

The term dual diagnosis has been coined to describe patients with coexistent mental illness and substance misuse problems (Carey *et al.*, 1991). Some mentally ill patients may self medicate their symptoms with illicit drugs and alcohol (Dixon *et al.*, 1990) and stimulant type drugs may be used by some patients receiving neuroleptic medication to counteract distressing extra-pyramidal side-effects (Schneider and Siris, 1987). With the recent closures of long-stay psychiatric institutions and an increasing emphasis on care and treatment in the community, mentally ill patients are perhaps more exposed to a range of licit and illicit drugs than previously. Furthermore, mentally ill people who have become socially isolated, may be drawn into a drug using subculture, which appears more attractive and less stigmatized for social interactions.

This chapter will describe the nature and extent of mental health problems associated with substance misuse, and identify key features that might help the addiction nurse to distinguish between primary and secondary psychiatric disorders. It will also address the important treatment issues and implications for management illustrated further by a case vignette.

MENTAL HEALTH PROBLEMS AND SUBSTANCE MISUSE

Prevalence

Psychiatric disorders frequently overlap with substance misuse. A number of studies have shown a high prevalence of psychiatric features present in substance misusers and that substance misuse is a common problem among psychiatric patients. In their study, Glass and Jackson (1988) reviewed the discharge records on 43 000 patients treated in hospital over a 12-year period and of those patients with an 'alcoholic' diagnosis (9–11%) between 30–40% had an additional psychiatric diagnosis. Ross *et al.* (1988) using the diagnostic statistical manual DSM 111 criteria found over two thirds of patients referred to an addiction unit had a current psychiatric diagnosis, usually affective disorder, anxiety or antisocial personality. Similarly, Rieger and colleagues (1988) found that 71% of substance misusers also had a mental disorder. Earlier work carried out by Hall *et al.* (1979) found a high incidence (58%) of patients admitted to a psychiatric unit with a history of drug misuse.

Mental health problems

The chronic use and intoxication of drugs such as amphetamines, cocaine, cannabis, ecstacy and LSD can produce symptoms such as suspiciousness, agitation, emotional lability, paranoid delusions, perceptual distortions and hallucinations. However, these symptoms are also found in paranoid schizophrenia and may be exacerbated by certain illicit drugs (Smith and Hucker, 1994, Creighton *et al.*, 1991).

Skilled diagnosis may often be required to differentiate between a drug induced and functional psychosis (non-drug induced). Visual and tactile hallucinations have been found to be more common in the former whereas auditory hallucinations and persecutory delusions tend to be more characteristic of the latter (Ghodse, 1989). A key feature of amphetamine induced psychoses is the absence of confusion and disorientation as psychotic symptoms tend to occur in a setting of clear consciousness. Stereotyped or repetitive behaviour and 'picking' of the skin (parasitosis) are also common characteristics of stimulant related psychoses. Chronic intoxication from stimulant drugs may result in a hypomanic state with accompanying symptoms such as extreme restlessness, irritability, over-talkativeness and flight of ideas.

Perceptual disturbances including illusions and hallucinations, delusions, and seizures may occur following withdrawal from CNS depressants such as alcohol, benzodiazepines, barbiturates and chlormethiazole. Hallucinations are frequently of a visual and auditory nature. Alcoholic hallucinosis is a rare condition that may occur either during withdrawal or intoxication from alcohol and is characterized mainly by auditory hallucinations of a derogatory type. However, unlike delirium tremens where there is generalized confusion and disorientation, patients suffering from hallucinosis are usually oriented and not confused.

Depressive symptoms such as low mood, sleep disturbance, poor appetite and suicidal pre-occupation are commonly found among opiate and hypno-sedative drug misusers (including alcohol misusers) and may also follow stimulants withdrawal. However, in a number of clients these symptoms may persist long after detoxification, and in such clients the presence of an underlying depressive illness should be strongly suspected. Suicide and para-suicides are substantially higher among substance misusers than the general population (Murphy, 1988) and the mortality rate has been estimated to be 15% (Hawton, 1987).

Anxiety, panic attacks and phobic symptoms may be precipitated by the chronic use of benzodiazepines, stimulants, hallucinogens, cannabis and alcohol. These are particularly common during the course of alcohol and benzodiazepine with drawal, but in some patients may predate their substance misuse and will require specific psychological treatments. Irritability, restlessness and aggressive behaviour may result from either intoxication or withdrawal of these drugs and memory impairment is commonly associated with heavy use of CNS depressants. Wernicke's encephalopathy and Korsakoff's psychosis are two related conditio. that may occur following chronic alcohol misuse resulting in severe memory disturbances, mood changes and perceptual disturbances.

Nursing interventions

Assessment

Psychoactive substances act on the CNS and in so doing will affect changes in mood and thought. It is therefore important during the course of assessment to observe for any abnormal changes in mood, thinking and behaviour. All too often addiction nurses tend to regard the assessment of a client's mental condition to be the responsibility of a psychiatrist and may spend the entire interview focusing on details of drug use.

Failure to recognize psychiatric symptoms at an early stage will lead to ineffective treatment strategies, and may result in the worsening of the client's mental health problems. When there is evidence of signs and symptoms of mental health problems, the nurse should ask the client to elaborate on these and to relate them to the use of specific substances along with periods of intoxication, withdrawal or abstinence. This will help in distinguishing cause from effect and may aid the diagnostic process between a primary and secondary psychiatric disorder.

As already outlined, this relationship is not always easy to determine since clients may find it difficult to describe their symptoms in any logical sequence. However, the nurse could facilitate this process by getting clients to identify the onset, duration and severity of their symptoms. For example, in the case of an amphetamine user who complains of feeling depressed, it is important to identify whether such feelings predated their drug use or whether they persisted during periods of being drug free. Likewise for a client who experiences symptoms of anxiety and panicky feelings relating to the use of benzodiazepines, the addiction nurse would want to establish whether these occur during use, during withdrawal or prior to the onset of drug use.

A family history of psychiatric illness should raise the possibility of substance misuse being secondary to an underlying psychiatric disorder. In addition, the nurse should make an assessment of the client's pre-morbid personality and the degree of insight into the nature of his or her mental health problems.

Management

Having gained an understanding of the nature and severity of a client's mental health problems the nurse will be able to develop an appropriate care plan with the client that will help to alleviate psychological distress. For the client who is experiencing psychotic symptoms such as hallucinations, delusions and emotional lability, admission to hospital for monitoring and stabilization of his or her mental state should be facilitated.

In most cases a drug induced psychosis will resolve without medical intervention once the effects of the drug have worn off. Depending upon the duration and action of the drug used, this may take between 24 and 72 hours. In the case of an amphetamines related psychosis, if psychotic symptoms persist for longer than a week after negative urine tests, another primary psychiatric illness must be considered (Lishman, 1987). A cannabis induced psychoses may last longer as cannabis, which is lipid soluble, is metabolized and excreted more slowly from the body.

On admission, the client should be managed in a quiet part of the ward and kept away from any unnecessary stimulation. A calm and reassuring approach by the staff will help to alleviate symptoms such as anxiety, restlessness and agitation but in some cases medication may be required. Diazepam is effective in reducing agitation, irritability and sleeplessness. It also helps to prevent fits in clients undergoing withdrawal from CNS depressants including alcohol.

For the acutely ill psychotic client whose behaviour is disturbed and presents management problems, neuroleptic drugs such as chlorpromazine and haloperidol can be effective. However, care should be taken to minimize against neuroleptic induced side-effects by using the lowest optimum dose required for the shortest possible duration. Such prescribing safeguards are necessary since anti-Parkinsonian drugs such as kemadrin prescribed to reduce the side-effects of anti-psychotic medication are themselves prone to abuse by stimulant users (Pullen *et al.*, 1984).

Persistent anxiety and depressive symptoms following sedatives and stimulant withdrawal may be indicative of a pre-existing psychiatric disorder that will require specific treatments. Tricyclic antidepressant drugs such as desipramine have been found to be effective in depression following stimulant drug use. Clients experiencing mental health problems as a result of their substance misuse should be informed about the particular effects and complications different drugs may have on their mental state, and should be encouraged to abstain from these drugs if possible.

Social skills training, problem-solving skills, stress management and relaxation techniques are all useful interventions in helping clients to deal with situations in which illicit drug use may occur. In addition problems relating to unstable accommodation and unemployment would need to be addressed and the nurse should liaise with welfare agencies such as social services and housing associations on behalf of clients. Attendance at a mental health resource day centre will help unemployed clients to avoid boredom and drug using peers.

Case vignette

John is 23 years old and works as a chef in a famous restaurant. His parents separated when he was 14 years old and his mother was later admitted to a psychiatric unit with a 'nervous breakdown'. John began smoking cannabis intermittently after leaving school at 16 and also took ecstasy and amphetamines at the weekends. At the age of 18 he enlisted on a two year chef's training course at college. During this period John's use of cannabis and amphetamines increased to daily use and he continued to take them with LSD, and ecstasy at weekend raves.

The police were called to the restaurant where John worked one evening after staff had found him in a disturbed state. He was brandishing a knife and accusing his work colleagues of trying to poison him. John was admitted to hospital in an agitated and restless state and he now directed his paranoid ideas towards the nursing staff accusing them of putting poison into his tea. He was also picking at his skin and complaining of flying insects in the ward.

Nursing Intervention

John was managed in a quiet part of the ward as he was easily distracted and got into arguments with other patients. He needed constant reassurance from staff that he was in hospital because he was unwell and that the nurses were there to help him get better. He seemed to respond to this and appeared less suspicious with nurses with whom he was familiar. He was prescribed diazepam at night to help his sleeplessness and his mental condition improved over the next two days.

His paranoid ideas disappeared and he began socializing with other patients on the ward. He was encouraged to participate in the various therapeutic activities on the ward such as anxiety and stress management sessions and drugs educational groups. The results from a drug screen carried out at the time of his admission confirmed the presence of amphetamines and cannabis. John was informed that his condition was drug related and that his symptoms could reoccur should he return to illicit drug use. He was subsequently discharged from hospital symptom free and was followed-up by a community psychiatric nurse (CPN). He was encouraged to avoid former drug using peers and to pursue other recreational interests.

Problems and issues

Where a psychiatric disorder and substance misuse co-exist, it is often difficult to distinguish between cause and effect. For example, in the case of an alcohol dependent client who presents with depressive symptoms, four possible explanations could be considered. First, that dependence on alcohol is primarily related to an underlying depression which predates the onset of heavy drinking. Second, that the depression is due to the depressant effects of alcohol on the brain. Third, that the client has become depressed as a result of the negative psychosocial consequences associated with alcohol abuse and fourth a psychiatric disorder and substance use disorders may occur independently of each other.

This task of diagnosis is further complicated by the fact that many substance misusers are using a wide variety of psychoactive substances. Clients may not be able to understand the nature of the symptoms they experience or adequately to describe them in a way that enables the nurse to differentiate between a primary and secondary mental disorder. This distinction is not just of theoretical interest but has practical importance in developing an effective treatment and management plan for the client experiencing distressing mental health symptoms. Because of their close involvement with clients and ability to engage them in a trusting therapeutic relationship, nurses are in a unique position closely to observe and monitor symptoms and behaviour.

It has been suggested by Minkoff (1989) that dual diagnosis patients (i.e. patients with drug and alcohol problems secondary to a psychiatric illness) are best treated by the general psychiatric services. Such patients may find specialist drug and alcohol services too confrontational and stress provoking. Also in a group situation, dual diagnosis patients may be pressurized by other clients to abstain from prescribed medication and this could result in a deterioration of their mental condition. However, since clients experiencing psychiatric symptoms associated with substance misuse will present in different treatment settings, services should adopt a flexible response to ensure that prompt and effective help is provided.

In some cases it may be necessary to link up with the general psychiatric services and to develop a shared care approach with the substance misuse nurse acting as a specialist resource to generic health workers. Compliance with taking prescribed medication has been shown to be poor in mentally ill clients with substance misuse problems (Pristach and Smith, 1990) and the involvement of a CPN can help to increase clients' compliance with taking medication as well as monitoring mental health symptoms. It also helps to intervene early and facilitate access to treatment in the event of relapse.

CONCLUSION

The co-existence of substance misuse and mental health problems presents great challenges for clinicians and requires skilled assessment and intervention. These clients tend to have complex health and social needs in addition to their substance misuse problems and a failure to recognize these can lead to ineffective treatment outcomes. Because of the nature of their interaction with patients and a holistic approach to practice, nurses can make a significant contribution to the recognition and treatment of the substance misuser with mental health problems.

Helping clients to understand the nature of their symptoms and the effects various drugs and alcohol might have on their mental state should be undertaken throughout the treatment process. This is of particular importance since many clients may be tempted to return to substance misuse after their symptoms have subsided. In addition, those clients with a primary mental illness and who are receiving psychiatric medication such as antidepressants or neuroleptics, should be encouraged to take these and to keep their follow up appointments. A friendly letter, home visit or telephone call to remind some clients of their appointments may improve attendance rates by giving them a sense of importance and a feeling that someone really cares. Obviously clinical judgement and sensitivity is required in striking a balance between the need to provide personal responsibility and avoiding a 'spoon-fed' approach. However, some clients especially those with chaotic and disorganized lifestyles do respond to a friendly and flexible approach and maximizing their compliance with treatment could well avert later crises.

REFERENCES

Carey, M.P., Carey, K.B. and Meisler, A.W. (1991) Psychiatric symptoms in mentally ill chemical abusers. *Journal of Nervous and Mental Diseases*, **179**(3), 136–38.

Creighton, F. G., Black, D.L. and Hyde, C.E. (1991) 'Ecstasy' psychosis and flashbacks. *British Journal of Psychiatry*, **159**, 713–15.

Dixon, L., Haas, J., Weiden, P. *et al.* (1990) Acute effects of drug abuse in schizophrenic patients: clinical observation and patients' self reports. *Schizophrenia Bulletin*, **16**(1), 69–79.

Glass, I.B. and Jackson, P. (1988) Maudsley Hospital Survey: prevalence of alcohol problems and other psychiatric disorders in a hospital population. *British Journal of Addiction*, **83**(9), 1105–11.

Ghodse, H. (1989) *Drugs and Addictive Behaviour: A Guide To Treatment*, Blackwell Scientific Publications, Oxford.

Hall, R.C.W., Stickney, S.K., Gardener, E.R. *et al.* (1979) Relationship of psychiatric illness to drug use. *Journal of Psychedelic Drugs*, **11**(4), 337–42.

Hawton, K. (1987) Assessment of suicide risk. *British Journal of Psychiatry*, **150**, 52–3.

Lishman, W.A. (1987) *Organic Psychiatry*, 2nd ed, Blackwell Scientific Publications, Oxford.

Minkoff, K. (1989) Integrated treatment models of dual diagnosis of psychosis and addiction. *Hospital Community Psychiatry*, **40**(10), 1031–6

Murphy, G.E. (1988) Suicide and substance abuse. *Archives of General Psychiatry*, **45**, 593–594.

Pristach, C.A. and Smith, C.M. (1990) Medication compliance and substance abuse among schizophrenic patients. *Hospital Community Psychiatry*, **41**(12), 1345–48.

Pullen, G.P., Best, M.R. and Maguire, J. (1984) Anticholinergic drug abuse: a common problem? *British Medical Journal*, **289**(6445), 612–13.

Rieger, D.A., Boyd, J.H., Burke, J.D. *et al.* (1988) One-month prevalence of mental disorders in the United States. *Archives of General Psychiatry*, **45**(11), 977–86.

Ross, H.E., Glaser, F.B., Stiasny, S. *et al.* (1988) Sex differences in the prevalence of psychiatric disorders in patients with alcohol and drug problems. *British Journal of Addiction*, **83**(10), 1179–92.

Schneider, F.R. and Siris, S.D. (1987) A review of psychoactive substance use and abuse in schizophrenia: patterns of drug choice. *Journal of Nervous Mental Disorders*, **175**(11), 641–52.

Smith, J. and Hucker, S. (1994) Schizophrenia and substance abuse. British Journal of Psychiatry, **165**, 13–21.

PART FOUR
Prevention, health education and collaboration

Addiction nursing: a new direction in prevention

18

Elizabeth McShane

INTRODUCTION

Licit and illicit substance use and misuse remain the largest cause of preventable morbidity and mortality in the UK. The importance of early recognition and intervention in addictive substance use is undisputed. Primary healthcare teams are well placed to offer screening and early intervention. Patients trust their doctor's advice and, as about 90% of the practice population visit the surgery within any three-year period, there are many opportunities to influence a large number of patients (Glanz and Taylor,1986; Abed and Neira-Munoz, 1990). Yet development of training for members of the primary health care staff in the relevant skills has been slow. Addiction Prevention Counselling is a new community based initiative which attempts to address the issue of substance misuse at an early stage in the career of a potential substance misuser. This approach deals with individuals with alcohol and illicit substance misuse problems as well as smoking and over the counter preparations.

In this chapter the concept of addiction prevention in primary care is introduced and the role of the addiction prevention counsellor is examined. The development of addiction prevention and its aims is addressed. In addition the benefits to clients and those involved in treating them in the primary care setting are identified.

DEVELOPMENT OF ADDICTION PREVENTION IN PRIMARY CARE PROGRAMMES

The concept of prevention in the primary care setting is not new, but the establishment of The Addiction Prevention in Primary Care Programme (APC) with specialist interest in substance use and misuse is the first of its kind in the UK (Saunders *et al.*, 1995; Ghodse *et al.*, 1995). The programme has served as the prototype for other such services. It embraces the concepts of early identification and intervention and does not limit itself to any one aspect of drug use and misuse. It reflects the transition from ward based healthcare delivery to community based care, and its focus also reflects the targets as laid down in *The Health of the Nation document* (Department of Health, 1992). What is most promising is that the project deals with all members of the primary health care team and supports the view that good projects in physical health and mental health do not necessarily have to be carried out by psychiatric trained staff or those based in a mental health setting and are not restricted to one particular professional group.

The development of the programme is, in effect, the result of the massive upheaval in patient care. These changes stem from the research evidence into cost effective treatment options available to patients. Evaluation studies have compared the effectiveness of different types of detoxification services. These evaluation data have been and remain contentious, mainly because it is difficult to make direct comparisons between studies of detoxification. Many have different aims and no one service will suit all clients.

Aims of APC programmes

The APC programme aims to facilitate primary healthcare staff in the early recognition of and intervention in the problems associated with substance use and misuse. The project covers all classes of psychoactive substances including social drugs (e.g. alcohol and tobacco), licit substances (e.g. benzodiazepines and solvents) and illicit drugs (e.g. cannabis, and ecstasy). The main aim of the programme is to equip primary healthcare staff with the necessary skills, knowledge and confidence to enable them to work effectively in this field.

Role of the addiction counsellor

The counsellors work with practice staff to offer a surgery based counselling service to patients at an early stage of problem or hazardous substance use/misuse. They can establish a smoking cessation and/or other substance misuse clinics or programmes as appropriate. Counsellors offer the practice one clinical session a week for a period of three to five months before handing over the clinical work to surgery staff they have trained and to whom they offer ongoing support. In this aspect we do not train practice staff to become counsellors. Our aim is to facilitate primary healthcare staff to utilize counselling and communication skills more effectively when assessing patients' level of substance use/misuse and to negotiate a treatment plan.

How does an addiction prevention counsellor work?

Predominantly the role is patient centred, to ensure that the treatment process is a positive experience for the patient. This is particularly important as the programme targets individuals who have not had treatment previously for smoking, drinking or illicit drug use. Negative experiences will discourage patients from returning to their GP or practice nurse (PN). Patient goal setting is therefore vital. The underpinning principles of patient treatment matching, a brief intervention and motivational interviewing in the APCs experience increase the likelihood of a successful treatment outcome.

Goal setting and outcome

When working with patients in general practice the setting of goals is very much directed by the patients themselves. If patients then achieve their goals this is considered a successful outcome. These goals are not always what counsellors might consider the ideal. For example, the counsellor might consider that total cessation of smoking or drinking is an ideal goal. However, unless this coincides with the patient view the probability of success is reduced. Clients who misuse psychoactive substances tend not to view the consequences in the long term. In contemplating cessation smoking they will want to know how they will feel after one week and not necessarily after one year. However, if the patient experiences success in any form they are more likely to enter into new goal setting.

Patient treatment matching

Working in general practice, it is also common to come into contact with patients who have had previous attempts at detoxification from a variety of substances. In many cases, opiate detoxification is self managed and occurs without formal assistance (Gossop *et al.*, 1991). It is clear that no one particular treatment approach will suit all who use and potentially misuse drugs. Consequently much research is now focused on whether treatment outcomes can be improved by systematically matching patients according to certain characteristics with the treatment approach that is potentially most effective.

The data on patterns of substance use obtained by the APC indicate the patient's presenting problem and does not necessarily give the total picture of the individual's substance use. For example, the patient presenting as a smoker who also uses cannabis would be recorded as a 'smoker'. Accurate screening of total drug use is an important factor in designing an effective treatment plan whether or not the patient regards their illicit drug use as problematic. Providing patients with a range of options increases their sense of ownership and personal responsibility. Initially, it is sometimes necessary to steer patients in the direction of less intensive treatments. If the patient is unsuccessful in the beginning you have not exhausted the range of treatments available.

Brief intervention

Underpinning much of the work of the APC is that of The Brief Intervention Approach. While there is no generally accepted definition of a brief intervention there are common elements which the APCs follow. The number of sessions varies between 8–10 and are of 10–20 minutes duration. The content of these sessions usually involves feedback to the patients about personal risk or impairment that has resulted from their substance use, the emphasis being on the patients' role or responsibility for change. This is followed by clear advice to change and the individual is given accurate information on what is available. There is no one absolute therapeutic stance adopted by the APCs but empathy underpins the counselling style. Within the team itself the approach is cognitive/behavioural and psychodynamic.

Motivational Interviewing

Motivational Interviewing (MI) is based on the work of Prochaska and Di Clemente (1983) and, as a therapeutic intervention, is widely accepted as one of the most useful models of change in this field. Thus, in our work motivation is considered to be a pre-condition for treatment. Previous models tend to define motivation in terms of individual characteristics and patients are either motivated or not. Lack of motivation is simplistically explained in terms of failure to comply or to continue in treatment. In Prochaska and Di Clemente's model, motivation is reflected in what the individual does. It involves recognizing a problem, identifying a way to change and then beginning, continuing and complying with change strategies (Miller and Heather, 1986).

Recognition and early identification

Surveys reveal that while GPs and practice nurses recognize the value in asking patients about their alcohol consumption, they are reluctant to intervene (Anderson, 1985; 1993). There are a number of possible explanations for this. First, these may reflect conventional beliefs and sensitivities regarding the nature of alcohol and its treatment. Second, GPs are increasingly being encouraged to undertake a variety of secondary prevention activities and they may assign a low priority status to alcohol issues when faced with increasing demands and workload. Finally, there are concerns about addressing health issues with patients who are not necessarily seeking help for alcohol-related problems.

The WHOs study (Babor and Grant, 1992) found that patients were easier to recruit in primary care settings than in hospital or the workplace. In a UK study involving 47 general practices, Wallace *et al.* (1988) reported a 21% reduction in alcohol consumption as a result of simple advice and information delivered by GPs. Were this activity carried out by every GP in the country it could reduce the alcohol consumption of 250 000 men and 67 000 women to moderate levels.

According to a review of the literature published in the *Effective Health Care Bulletin* (Nuffield Institute for Health, 1993), the opportunistic screening of patients in the primary care setting and the delivery of a brief intervention is economical, costing around £20 per patient. With the focus on achieving Health of the Nation targets, this information should be of great interest to directors of public health and purchasers of health services. While these findings are encouraging, research is still needed to determine the durability of the effects of brief intervention and the cumulative success rates of applying brief interventions routinely in primary practice. More information is needed on the nature and extent of health gains following intervention in primary care, and on the effectiveness of screening and intervention when delivered by the practice nurse. It has been suggested by Duckert (1994) that training might be better undertaken by those who are skilled in encouraging people to make lifestyle changes such as weight reduction and smoking cessation experts rather than traditional alcohol experts working at a tertiary level.

ESTABLISHING A SERVICE FOR SUBSTANCE USERS/MISUSERS

There are many benefits in establishing a service for substance users/misusers.

- Benefits to the client.
  The service is client centred so that individuals can set their own goals and can self-refer. They can choose from a range of options, and can decide that this is not the 'right time' and can approach the service later. There is a reduction in waiting time, and the service is non-stigmatizing.

- Benefits to the GP.
  The effectiveness of early and brief intervention strategies in reducing smoking and harmful drug use has been well documented particularly with regard to long-term treatment costs associated with substance misuse e.g. coronary heart disease. These strategies reduce the pressure on appointments, as heavy alcohol users, for example, tend to use their GP twice as much as other patients. In single-handed practices, GPs receive regular ongoing feedback about their patients.

- Benefits to the practice nurse and primary healthcare staff.
  Sometimes it is not easy to see the benefits. There are the usual concerns about the amount of additional time that might be taken up with patients and not having the necessary skills. Also, it is important to acknowledge their own stereotypes with regard to substance users/misusers in general. Primary healthcare staff receive training and this can be tailored to meet individuals' needs. There is ongoing follow-up and staff can contact the APC staff at any time. Thus, there is the development of skills and confidence.

- Benefits to the APC.
  The service enables the nurse to become an autonomous practitioner in his/her own right. As this is a relatively new role for nurses in general practice it fulfils, in many aspects, Castledine's (1982) definition of the clinical nurse specialist as a 'trained nurse with additional nursing education who has been carrying out direct clinical nursing practice with specific patients in a specific branch of nursing'. The role of an APC is not exclusive to nursing as the team comprises a counsellor, a nurse and a social worker. Since there is increasing demand from the public for better services and care, the handing over from doctors to nurses specific areas of care and skills previously considered the domain of medicine can increase efficiency.

Working with smokers

In order to clarify some of the work of the addiction nurse this section will focus on the work that we do with people who smoke. This is for two main reasons. First, they present most often to their GP or practice nurse for advice and information on how to stop smoking. Second, when setting up a substance use/misuse service in general practice one is often met with resistance. GPs will have the erroneous view that, through establishing such a service, this will attract the 'wrong sort' or a very problematic opiate using patient group. By reminding GPs and practice nurses of the banding requirements, focusing on the smoker to begin with provides a way into the general practice setting. Initially, GPs may state that they do not have any long-term tranquillizer users and that they rarely see an alcohol problem. The experience of the APC is that after having been at the surgery for a period of time tranquillizer and alcohol users will appear on the appointments list.

Individuals who consult their GP or practice nurse about their smoking behaviour will by and large have been smoking for some time. It is not unusual for an individual to have been smoking since early childhood. They are often familiar with most strategies for smoking cessation e.g. nicotine replacement products, non nicotine replacement products, hypnosis, acupuncture, etc. Many will have had a history of unsuccessful attempts at stopping, some of which may have been associated with a life threatening illness or because a partner has stopped. These issues in themselves can make it difficult to view positively or hopefully another attempt at stopping.

Assessment

In assessing a smoker it is necessary to clarify at the outset helpful and hindering factors that may lead to a successful outcome. Do they want to stop or have they been sent by their practice nurse, GP, wife, husband or because they are having to undergo surgery? If the patient does not want to stop then alerting them to the health risks and providing them with information to read is sometimes the most appropriate course of action. Follow-up at a later date with regard to smoking might identify individuals who are now ready to stop for themselves. If they want to stop they ask when do they have their first cigarette of the day. This gives the counsellor an indication of the level of dependence. Other questions that might be asked at the assessment include:

- how many do they smoke and what brand of cigarette do they use;
- do they smoke other substances e.g. cannabis (it will not be possible for many to stop smoking and to continue smoking cannabis);
- does their partner smoke (if the answer is yes then this will also affect their chances of success) – perhaps if both partners are interested in giving up then seeing them together may prove more successful;
- have they ever stopped before (if yes for how long) – what precipitated that attempt and what factors resulted in relapse focusing on what helped the individual to stay off. Identifying high risk areas provides a basis for relapse planning (Marlatt and George, 1984).

Asking the client what they want to achieve. Is it simply to cut down or to stop altogether? At this point one may say that any level of cigarette smoking is damaging to ones health. In the experience of the APC it is wise and prudent to work with the patients' goals when first in contact. What often emerges is that, although the client may be successful in cutting down, staying at the reduced level proves more problematic than first anticipated. The patient is then more open to consider total cessation.

Interventions

A typical programme consists of setting a 'stop' date usually about four weeks ahead. During the intervening weeks the client identifies coping strategies and works towards the 'stop' date. Sometimes the individual will alter the nicotine and tar level though not necessarily the amount smoked. Nicotine replacement products are discussed and some patients are willing to try nicotine patches to see how they will cope. A low level nicotine patch is suggested initially to allow room for a higher level patch to be used. Some people do not alter their smoking behaviour at all when they are working towards their stop date. Other options about smoking cessation groups are discussed. Some patients are willing to enter into a smoking cessation group for the additional support. Setting up smoking cessation groups is not always easy. It is more likely if there are large numbers of patients looking to stop at the same time particularly before or just after the new year. The initial resolve following over indulgence needs to be monitored. Having arrived at the stop date follow-up sessions are planned. This has proved to be helpful to patients as they value the additional support. Though not always successful the treatment contact is seen as positive and most patients are willing to look at their smoking again at a later date. It is a difficult area but the same principles apply to other drugs of misuse.

CONCLUSION

It is the experience of the APC that offering a clinical service in general practice leads to a heightened awareness of substance misuse problems and earlier intervention. This supports the viability of promoting early intervention into substance misuse through offering a practice based service. The programme uses a horizontal approach to sharing expertise. The counsellor is viewed as a peer and this has proved more acceptable than formal instruction from someone viewed as a superior. The programme successfully bridges the interfaces between hospital based specialist services, the academic institution with its research and educational resources and primary healthcare which is the front-line for prevention strategies and risk reduction.

By working in general practice, the counsellors have developed a better understanding of the way in which GPs work and have adapted strategies to the working philosophies of individual practices. As a result, further developments in addiction prevention have been sensitive to the requirements of GPs and other practice staff. These include the publication of leaflets specifically aimed at helping patients and a series of 'How to help' cards, designed to assist professionals to intervene at an earlier stage of substance misuse.

It would be a wasted opportunity not to capitalize on the advantages offered by the general practice setting in which 90% of the practice population are seen within a three year period, and where there is a relatively low turnover in staff. Training practice staff to continue work after the APC has left is cost effective in the long term. More patients can be screened and assessed with the potential for intervening in a potential substance misusing career. The benefits cannot be ignored.

REFERENCES

Abed, R.T. and Neira-Munoz, E. (1990) A Survey of General Practitioners' opinion and attitude to drug addicts and addiction. *British Journal of Addiction*, **85**(1), 131–36.

Anderson, P. (1985) Managing alcohol problems in general practice. *British Medical Journal*, **290**(6485) 1873–1975

Anderson, P. (1993) Effective general practice of interventions for patients with harmful alcohol consumption. *British Journal of General Practice*, **43**(37), 386–89.

Babor, T.F., Ritson, E.B. and Hodgson, R.J. (1986). Alcohol Related Problems in the Primary Health Care Setting: a review of early intervention strategies. *British Journal of Addiction*, **81**(1), 23–46.

Babor, T.F. and Grant, H. (1992) *WHO Collaborating Investigators Project on Identification and Management of Alcohol – Related Problems*, WHO, Copenhagen.

Casteldine, G. (1982) Just like Topsy, the job grew ... development, future role and function of Clinical Nurse Specialists. *Nursing Mirror*, **155**(80), 48.

Department of Health (1992) *The Health of the Nation: A strategy for Health in England*, HMSO, London.

Duckert, F. (1994) Identification and management of alcohol problems in primary health-care. *Addiction*, **89**(6), 667–8.

Ghodse, A.H., McShane, E., Priestley, J.S. and Saunders, V.J. (1995) Addiction Prevention in Primary Care Programme Review 1993/1994. Centre for Addiction Studies, St George's Hospital Medical School.

Glanz, A. and Taylor, C. (1986) Findings of a National Survey of the role of General Practitioner in the treatment of Opiate Misuse: Extent of contact with opiate misusers. *British Medical Journal*, **293**(6546), 543–5.

Gossop, M., Battersby, M. and Strang, J. (1991) Self detoxification by opiate addicts: a preliminary investigation. *British Journal of Psychiatry*, **159**, 208–12.

Marlatt, G.A. and George, W.H. (1984) Relapse Prevention: introduction and overview of the model. *British Journal of Addiction*, **79**(3), 261–73.

Miller, W.R. and Heather, N. (1986) *Addictive Behaviours*, Plenum Press, New York.

Nuffield Institute for Health (1993) *Brief interventions and Alcohol Use*, Effective Health Care Bulletin, Number 7, University of Leeds, Leeds.

Prochaska, J.O. and DiClemente, C.C. (1983) Stages and processes of self change of smoking: Towards an integrative model of change. *Journal of Consulting and Clinical Psychology*, **51**(3), 390–95.

Saunders, V., McShane, E. and Priestley, J.S. (1995) Addiction Prevention in Primary Care. Substance Misuse Bulletin **8**(2), 8.

Wallace, P.G., Cutler, S. and Haines, A. (1988) Randomised controlled trial of general practitioner intervention in patients with excessive alcohol consumption. *British Medical Journal*, **297**(6649), 663–68.

19

Health education, prevention and harm-minimization

G.Hussein Rassool and Mike Gafoor

INTRODUCTION

Health education and prevention are increasingly important aspects of healthcare as the NHS reforms continue. The health and social costs incurred to the health-care system through the misuse of alcohol, tobacco smoking and other psychoactive substances have shifted public services towards more effective prevention programmes in substance use. The advent of HIV/AIDS has also influenced health and social policies and unveiled new prevention initiatives and challenges towards substance misuse.

The Ottawa Charter for Health Promotion (WHO, 1986) provides a valuable framework for preventive health intervention strategies for substance misuse. In the UK, there should be a proactive preventive policy reflecting the changing nature and extent of substance misuse. In addition, an integrated preventive policy covering alcohol, tobacco smoking, prescribed and illegal drugs, service provision and health education measures should be the hallmark of future policy development. The realization that some substance misusers engage in high risk behaviours, such as sharing of injecting equipment, having unsafe sex and of transmitting the HIV virus to the wider population, provided new impetus for the broad application of a harm-minimization approach in the substance misuse field.

This chapter aims to examine briefly the concept of health education, promotion and prevention, and outline various models and approaches to health education in the context of substance misuse. In addition, the concept and practice of harm-minimization and its implications for addiction nurses will be explored.

HEALTH EDUCATION AND HEALTH PROMOTION

There are several broad definitions of health education and health promotion and it is beyond the scope of this section to examine critically these concepts comprehensively. Examination of the concepts of health education and health promotion are covered more fully in the literature (Downie *et al.*, 1990; Tones, 1986; Ewles and Simnet, 1992; Tones and Tilford, 1994). The meaning of health education depends upon different ideologies, philosophies, approaches of education and models of health. According to Tones and Tilford (1994), health education is defined as 'any communication activity aimed at enhancing positive health and preventing or diminishing ill health in individuals and groups, through influencing the beliefs, attitudes and behaviour of those with power and of the community at large'. Thus, health education attempts to influence the attitudes, lifestyles and behaviour of individuals and the community by increasing their knowledge, skills and understanding of health and disease. Some writers have incorporated the concept of health education within the aegis of health promotion.

Maben and Macleod Clark (1995) propose a definition of health promotion that incorporates the concept of health education. Health promotion is seen as 'an attempt to improve the health status of an individual or community, and is also concerned with the prevention of disease ... At its broadest level it is concerned with the wider influences on health and therefore with the policy and legislative implications of these. Health education through information-giving, advice, support and skills training is part of, and necessary prerequisite to, health promotion'. However, in the context of this chapter, health education is referred to as an educational activity aimed at prevention of substance misuse and its sequelae in the general population, and in raising the awareness of the substance misusers towards positive health outcomes. It also incorporates the concept of harm-minimization.

PREVENTION

Prevention of substance use and misuse is everybody's business. It is a proactive process that utilizes an interdisciplinary approach designed to empower people with their resources constructively to confront stressful life situations (National Institute on Drug Abuse, 1980). The drive to minimize substance misuse and its sequelae has been along two main fronts: reducing the supply and demand. Strang and Farrell (1989) suggested that prevention programmes must be directed to encourage drug users to approach care services earlier in their drug using career rather than wait for the complications to appear before coming forward for help.

Traditionally, health education activities have been viewed as existing on three levels: primary; secondary; and tertiary prevention. This three-stage model has been modified by the Advisory Council on the Misuse of Drugs (ACMD, 1984) on the grounds that it was not comprehensive enough to cover all the elements of prevention policies. The ACMDs approach to prevention is based on meeting two basic criteria: reducing the risk of an individual engaging in substance misuse; and reducing the harm associated with substance misuse.

MODELS OF HEALTH EDUCATION

In the last decade, the trends in the care and management of substance misusers have shifted away from purely clinical and rehabilitative measures towards a positive health orientated approach. There are different models and approaches to health education and comprehensive examination of health education and health promotion concepts are covered in the literature: French (1990); Caplan and Holland (1990); Beattie (1991); Ewles and Simnett (1992); Naidoo and Willis (1994); Maben and Macleod Clarke (1995). This section will briefly examine five approaches to health education in relation to alcohol and drugs. The five different models are identified as: medical/public health model, educational model, behaviour change model, consumer's empowerment model and social change model.

The medical/public health model

This traditional model of health education is still widely dominant and is exemplified in the government's health strategy (Department of Health, 1992). This model focuses on primary prevention, that is, the prevention of illness and reduction of casualties. Its aims are to reduce both the premature mortality and morbidity among the substance use population. It involves, for example, screening and early recognition of alcohol/drug problems or immunization for hepatitis B and it may be treatment orientated. The medical model places both the cause and responsibility with the individual as 'victim blaming' and encourages compliance to a medical regimen. The major critique of this model is that the focus ignores the real sociopolitical roots of ill health (Tones and Tilford, 1994). It is argued that, in the past, this prescriptive model has influenced the medicalization of social problems.

Educational model

The aim of this model is to transmit health information and knowledge about substance misuse and to develop the necessary skills and coping strategies. This is based on the notion that the information provided will enable the individual to make decisions based on informed choices about the use of drugs, alcohol or tobacco smoking. In addition, this model may also provide individuals, through either one-to-one situation or group context, to explore their beliefs and attitudes towards their own health behaviours and lifestyles. The strength of this model is that it does not seek to impose the educator's own ideas and values or to persuade people to change their behaviour. However, inherent in this model, is the influence of value judgement of educational programmes and activities and, to some extent, to assume the individual's freedom of choice in the matter. It can still be criticized on the grounds that it focuses on the individual and takes little account of changing the socioeconomic environment which restricts the individual's freedom of choice (Ewles and Simnett, 1992).

Behaviour change model

The main focus of this model is to encourage individuals to change their health status by adopting new desirable patterns of health behaviours. That is, individuals have a responsibility to improve their health by changing their lifestyles regarding drug taking, eating, smoking, drinking or sexual behaviour. Many media campaigns, initiated by the Health Education Authority in England, regarding smoking, alcohol drinking or drug taking are orientated towards the behavioural change model. The main limitation of this model is that it disregards the interface between health behaviour and the socioeconomic determinants of health. Beside this, the healthcare professionals are expected to act as health experts to transmit information to effect the change in health behaviours of their clients. It is argued that 'it is most commonly an expert led, top down model, which reinforces the divide between the expert who knows how to improve health and the general public who need education and advice' (Naidoo and Willis, 1994).

Examples of health activities include education about controlled or sensible drinking, encouraging people to abstain from drugs, the promotion of anti-smoking attitudes or of promoting attitudes that drugtaking or smoking is anti-social. In addition, the promotion of patient education relating to safe sexual practices and about the rational use of psychoactive drugs (illicit, prescribed or over the counter drugs) are of prime importance.

Consumer's empowerment model

This model is consumer led and focuses on the individual or groups to identify their own concerns regarding specific health issues and their own health status. The role of the healthcare professional is to act as a facilitator and to 'empower' the individual or the community on health concerns and health education initiatives. Examples of this model include programmes relating to self-awareness, decision-making skills, value clarification and assertive skills.

In the context of drug and alcohol use/misuse, some of the community initiatives and self-help group movements have been initiated and led by parents' group (e.g. solvent abuse), the clients themselves (Alcohol Anonymous) or the Patients' Unions (Junkie Bond, Holland). This area of work is probably beyond the scope of most addiction nurses. However, addiction nurses in outreach work settings may have a specific remit to address health concerns or issues regarding substance misuse. The limitations of this model are due to limited financial resources, that they are sometimes 'led' by a medical expert, and may be timeconsuming or aimed at long-term outcomes. Also, there may be conflicts or differences of opinion about the use of specific models in terms of the needs among professionals, consumer's groups or the general public.

Social change model

This model focuses on the political, socioeconomic or structural determinants of health. It suggests implicitly that substance misuse is the result of socioeconomic factors and that the individual takes drugs or alcohol as a coping strategy. It has also been referred to as the 'political model of drug education or the radical model' (Tones and Tilford, 1994). This model, if applied to alcohol prevention, for example, would not only target the individual drinker but the powerful alcohol industry and the government. However, it is not clear whether raising the public's 'critical consciousness' of the activities of the alcohol industry and lobby would result in public support for more legislative controls such as higher taxation, statutory advertising and restrictions of licensing laws (Robinson and Baggot, 1985).

The contentious nature and political sensitivity of substance misuse are beyond the scope of professional practice for addiction nurses to adopt this model. However, it would be acceptable for healthcare professionals to raise awareness of health aspects of policy decisions. For instance, the recommended safe limits for alcohol intake, policy regarding the prescription of temazepam, the use of complementary therapies etc. Another criticism levelled at this model is that it may not be free of expert domination or the vested sociopolitical interest of health practitioners.

Table 19.1 summarizes the models, goals and health education's interventions in relation to drug and alcohol.

HEALTH EDUCATION IN ACTION

Prevention and health education of the general population towards the use and misuse of psychoactive substances are increasingly being recognized as part of the role of healthcare professionals and others (Department of Health, 1992; WHO/ICN, 1991). There is no single 'right' model of health education in the field of drug prevention and drug education. The model or models used by addiction nurses and other healthcare professionals in the prevention of substance misuse would depend on the ideology and professional practice of the 'health educator'. In addition, the health needs of the client, the context and setting, the client–worker relationship and the level of preventive health education will, undoubtedly, influence the choice of model(s). In the substance misuse field, a combination of approaches are utilized to complement other intervention strategies such as the harm-minimization approach.

Harm-minimization

Definition of concept

The concept of harm-minimization or harm-reduction may be viewed as the programmes and policies which attempt to reduce the harms associated with drug use

Table 19.1 Health education approaches to substance misuse

Models	Goals	Health education	Examples
Medical/public health	Reduction of morbidity and mortality	Prevention of ill health Clinical interventions	Early recognition, care, treatment and rehabilitation
Behaviour change	Change of life-style and behaviour	Media campaign Health Information: controlled drinking, safer drug use and safer sex.	Prevent non-smokers to start smoking Reduction of smokers Persuade smokers to stop Counselling Reducing or minimize ill effect or harm
Educational	Changing attitude Increase awareness and knowledge Developing skills in decision-making	Health information on smoking, drinking and drug-taking Learning coping skills and stress management	Information about effects of substance misuse and health-related problems
Social change	Enabling changes to health and social policies Bringing changes to the social environment Improvement in health and social equality in access to services and treatment interventions	Lobbying Political and social	Alcohol and drug policy in workplace Limit of marketing and advertising of psychoactive substances Labelling of alcoholic beverages

(Strang, 1993). A more comprehensive definition has been put forward by Watson (1991) who defines harm-reduction as 'the philosophical and practical development of strategies so that the outcomes of drug use are as safe as is situationally possible. It involves the provision of factual health information, resources, education, skills and the development of attitude change, in order, that the consequences of drug use for the users, the community and the culture have minimal negative impact'.

The concept of harm-minimization, therefore, goes beyond measures aimed at changing drug users' behaviours and involves wider societal changes such as legal sanctions, public attitudes and educational policies regarding drug use. It replaces the abstentionist thinking of the 1980s by recognizing that the use of psychoactive substances (licit and illicit) is widespread in society and that not all drug users will use drugs safely. Thus, approaches that aim to reduce the harms associated with drug use are more pragmatic and realistic.

Changes in policy

The term harm-minimization became accepted into the UK substance misuse vernacular in the mid 1980s as public concerns increased over the need to contain the spread of HIV infection among injecting drug users. In practice, clinicians in the drugs field had been quietly adopting harm-minimization strategies for many years, for example, with methadone maintenance and injectable prescribing. However, the concept was formally recognized as a policy framework for drug services with the ACMD (1988) report which set new priorities for working with drug users with its unambiguous statement that 'HIV is a greater threat to public and individual health than drug misuse ... services which aim to minimize HIV risk behaviour by all available means should take precedence in development plans'. This marked a major shift in policy thinking. The ACMD (1988) further recommended that services 'should adopt a hierarchy of goals in dealing with drug users' which should include:

- cessation of sharing injecting equipment;
- the move from injectable to oral drug use;
- decrease in drug use;
- abstinence.

Other sub-goals were later added to the hierarchy such as:

- cleaning injecting equipment before sharing;
- reducing the number of people with whom injecting equipment is shared;
- switching from illicit to prescribed drugs.

Drug services which had hitherto adopted different approaches to policy and practice were now in broad agreement that a harm-minimization approach was the most pragmatic response in curtailing the spread of HIV infection among drug users and to the wider community. According to Stimson (1990) the arrival of HIV/AIDS epidemic has had the effect of simplifying the debate in the muddled world of drug policy.

Seemingly overnight, protracted debates concerning issues, such as maintenance or abstinence and injectables or oral drugs, that had dogged the drugs field for many years began to fade away. Politicians, educationalists and community groups, previously committed to abstinence oriented campaigns (e.g. 'Just Say No'), were now calling for harm-minimization strategies. Drug workers are now being asked to abandon efforts to 'cure' addiction and to concentrate on reaching the harm associated with drug misuse.

A wide range of strategies is needed to address these harms some of which are described in chapter 6. Briefly, these involve the distribution of sterile injecting equipment and condoms, and providing HIV education to drug users. In addition, drug services have adopted more flexible prescribing policies and have lowered the threshold for treatment entry to attract those drug users not currently in touch with services.

In the alcohol field the concept of harm-free drinking was established with the publication of research showing that drinking behaviour could be modified (Heather and Robertson, 1989) and the issuing of the government's guidelines on sensible drinking (DHSS, 1981). As in the drugs field, a re-conceptualizing of alcohol problems away from an abstentionist and specialist framework in favour of public health and generalist model had already taken place. So what are the implications of health education and harm-minimization for addiction nurses?

Implications for addiction nurses

Addiction nurses have a key role in health education, promotion of health and the reduction of health risks in clients misusing psychoactive substances. Part of the role includes acting as a promoter of health (to campaign for policy and legislation to reduce the demands for psychoactive substances) and educator in teaching and providing health information on substance use and misuse to clients and the public.

Health teaching includes both knowledge and skills in dealing with problems associated with general health, drug/alcohol-related problems and coping strategies. Addiction nurses can make an impact on the general health of the client group in the promotion of adequate nutrition, exercise, safer sex, safer drug use, problem-solving and relapse prevention skills. The promotion of safer sex practices and safer drug use is seen as a high priority with hepatitis B and the advent of HIV infection. Many substance misusers are polydrug users with a high prevalence of tobacco smoking. Therefore, health education and promotion should also be targeted towards tobacco smoking and its health risks, and there should be the provision of smoking cessation clinics.

Over the past decade, many of the innovative clinical developments in the addiction field have been nurse led, for example low threshold methadone programmes, satellite clinics for homeless substance misusers, and HIV prevention work with street prostitutes. It is important that addiction nurses continue to play an active role in the future developments of both HIV and primary drug prevention initiatives as these two aims are not mutually exclusive. One of the central tenets of the Health of the Nation's document (Department of Health, 1992) is the need for healthy alliances in order to facilitate the co-ordination, integration and effective delivery of services (see chapter 20). Addiction nurses have developed particular skills in networking and service planning over the years and they should make sure that the competitive nature of the NHS reforms does not restrict inter-agency collaboration or inhibit new and imaginative initiatives. They should ensure that their views and ideas are conveyed to purchasers and service managers and that the newly established drug reference groups provide an important channel of communication.

The role of harm-minimization in primary and secondary educational programmes for young people who use drugs remains a contentious issue, although such an approach is fully accepted for work with alcohol. Many teachers, parents, and school governors fear that a drug harm-minimization approach might encourage drug use among those who might not otherwise have tried drugs. However, it is argued that drug use is an integral part of our society and experimenting with drugs is within the norms of adolescent behaviour (Irwin, 1989). As a result an educational approach that focuses on maximizing health and minimizing harm is more realistic and may be preferable to an abstinent oriented approach for some individuals. Furthermore, a prevention approach that makes an artificial distinction between licit and illicit psychoactive substances is likely to lack credibility with young people.

Addiction nurses with their specialist training and professional background have a crucial role in devising and implementing harm-minimization training programmes for teachers, parents, youth workers and other community groups involved in working with young people. Such programmes should include the physical and psychological effects of psychoactive substances, combined effects of multiple drugtaking, safer methods of drugtaking, stress management techniques and where to obtain help for substance misuse problems. In addition, addiction nurses have a role in the targeting of high risk subgroups, e.g. young offenders, for prevention strategies and helping to change the subcultural norms of drugtaking by involving peer groups as 'change agents'.

REFERENCES

Advisory Council on the Misuse of Drugs (1984) *Prevention*, HMSO, London.

Advisory Council on the Misuse of Drugs (1988) *AIDS and Drug Misuse Report: Part 1*, HMSO, London.

Beattie, A. (1991) Knowledge and control in health promotion: a test case for social policy and social theory, in *The Sociology of the Health Service* (eds J. Cabe, M. Calnan and M. Bury), Routledge, London.

Caplan, R. and Holland, R. (1990) Rethinking health education theory. *Health Education Journal*, **49**(1), 10–2.

Department of Health (1992) *The Health of the Nation. A Strategy for England*, HMSO, London.

DHSS (1981) *Drinking Sensibly*, HMSO, London.

Downie, R.S., Fyfe, C. and Tannahill, A. (1990) *Health Promotion. Models and Values*, Oxford University Press, Oxford.

Ewles, L. and Simnett, I. (1992) *Promoting Health*, Scutari Press, London.

French, J. (1990) Models of health education and promotion, *Health Education Journal*, **49**(1), 7–10.

Heather, N. and Robertson, I. (1989) *Problem Drinking*, 2nd edn, Oxford University Press, Oxford.

Irwin, C.E. (1989) Risk-taking behaviours in the adolescent patient: are they impulsive? *Paediatric Annals*, **18**, 122–3.

Maben, J. and Macleod Clarke, J.(1995) *Health promotion: a conceptual analysis. Journal of Advanced Nursing*, **22**(6), 1158–65.

Naidoo, J. and Willis, J. (1994) *Health Promotion: Foundations for practice*, Balliere Tindall, London.

National Institute of Drug Abuse (1980) The development approach to preventing problem dependencies, in *Community-based prevention specialist: Participant manual* (eds H.S. Glenn and J.W. Warner), NIDA, Rockville, MD, pp. 133–53.

Robinson, Y. and Baggott, R. (1985) Health Education and Prevention of Alcohol Problems. *Health Education Journal*, **44**(4), 493–95.

Stimson, G.V. (1990) Revising policy and practice: new ideas about the drugs problem, in *Aids and Drugs Misuse: The challenge for policy and practice in the 1990s* (eds J. Strang and G.V. Stimson), Routledge, London.

Strang, J. and Farrell, M. (1989) HIV and drug misuse: forcing the process of change. *Current Opinion in Psychiatry*, **2**, 402–7.

Strang, J. (1993) Drug use and harm reduction: responding to the challenge, in *Psychoactive Drugs and Harm Reduction: From Faith to Science* (eds N. Heather *et al.*), Wurr Publishers, London.

Tones, K. (1986) Preventing Drug Misuse: the case for breadth, balance and coherence. *Health Education Journal*, **45**(4), 223–30.

Tones, K. and Tilford, S. (1994) *Health Education, Effectiveness, Efficiency and Equity*, 2nd ed, Chapman and Hall, London.

Watson, M. (1991) Harm reduction – why do it? *International Journal on Drug Policy*, **2**(5), 13–5.

WHO (1986) *Ottawa Charter for Health Promotion*, WHO and Health and Welfare, Ottawa, Ontario.

World Health Organization/International Council of Nurses (1991) *Roles of the Nurse in relation to Substance Misuse*, ICN, Geneva.

20 | Interprofessional collaboration in addiction nursing

Olive McKeown

INTRODUCTION

The term 'Interprofessional Collaboration' has of late become a 'buzz word' in health and social care. The general pattern of healthcare reforms, most notably the shift from hospital and institutional care to community care has demanded more collaborative working among all health and social care professionals. Furthermore, specific health policies such as The Health of the Nation document (Department of Health, 1992) and *Tackling Drugs Together* (1995) have intensified the demand to collaborate and to work in partnership in an endeavour to operationalize these policies and reforms. Over the last few years, in response to the changes in health and social policy there has been an emergence of several new academic courses, professional journals and networking groups which aim to educate, guide and support health and social care staff in adjusting to their changing roles.

Nowhere, has the need for partnership and collaboration been greater than in the field of substance misuse. Addiction nurses have a particularly complex role, insofar as they deal with clients who present with wide-ranging and interrelated health and social needs. The nursing and clinical interventions commonly addressed from a social, psychological, legal and health perspective, guarantee that nurses frequently establish professional links with other relevant social, health and probation staff. This approach is not a new phenomenon for nurses working in substance misuse, but there is now an increased impetus to develop collaborative practices which are in line with recent policy initiatives.

The aim of this chapter is to explore the key issues facing addiction nurses with regard to interprofessional practice. This will be examined from a theoretical, practical and educational perspective: conflicts, challenges and barriers will be explored, and factors which may impede or enhance collaboration are discussed. Different approaches that address or overcome the problems are proposed.

TERMINOLOGY AND DEFINITIONS

Several terms are frequently used interchangeably, all essentially denoting the concept of interprofessional collaboration. For example, interprofessional co-operation, interprofessional working, partnership in care, inter-agency co-operation, health alliances, liaison, interdisciplinary working/teamwork, multidisciplinary teamwork or multiprofessional work. However, the precise meanings of these terms differ, and there is a trend for certain sections of health and welfare organizations to gravitate towards the use of particular terminology, e.g. the term 'inter-agency' seems to be referred to predominantly by social/welfare professionals and the 'partnership' is the one commonly utilized within recent health policy documentation.

Smoyak (1977) argues that a professional partnership only truly exists where there is joint decision-making and joint action. She states that 'combined action of involved professionals is the guiding framework of joint practice'. Ghodse (1995) defines 'partnership' as 'an association between a number of individuals, groups and agencies to pursue a common goal'. The essence of this definition is identical to Smoyak's, as the notion of 'a common goal' implicitly suggests that there is joint decision-making, while partnership refers to a cohesive form of joint working. Cartlidge (1987) describes 'collaboration' as existing at five different levels or stages, and the higher the stage, the greater the degree of collaboration. Cartlidge has formulated a taxonomy of collaboration as follows:

- isolation – members never meet, talk or write to each other;
- encounter – members who encounter or correspond with others but do not interact meaningfully;
- communication – members whose encounters or correspondence include the transference of information;
- collaboration between two agents – members who act sympathetically on shared formation, participate in joint working and share general objectives;
- collaboration throughout – organizations where the work of all members is fully integrated.

Health and social policy documentation relating to substance misuse issues commonly refer to 'partnership' which, within the framework of Cartlidge's taxonomy, denotes a high degree of collaborative practice.

HEALTH POLICY

The Health of the Nation document and *Tackling Drugs Together*, both government White Papers, represent the most recent and perhaps most important government initiatives in providing an impetus to interprofessional working in the substance misuse field. The document emphasizes that it is important for organizations and individuals 'to come together' to help improve health, that is to form 'healthy alliances'. The role of establishments such as 'healthy schools', 'healthy hospitals', 'healthy work places' etc. is regarded as an important means of contributing to a healthier general environment. Addiction nurses should grasp every opportunity to contribute to the establishment of improved alliances. This may take the form of offering advice and information as requested to individuals, groups or agencies. Addiction nurses may need to organize group discussions as well as establish educational groups for nurses and others. They may assist in the formulation of policies in response to substance misuse problems.

The recent publication of *Tackling Drugs Together: A Strategy For England 1995–1998*, sets out the government's strategy to tackle the drugs problem in England over the next few years. It sets clear national priorities, objectives and timetables, and creates a basis for action at community level. The government's commitment to reduce illegal drug demand through prevention, education and law enforcement is clearly stated. Within the introduction to the White Paper it is recommended that 'Effective partnership to protect individuals and communities is the foundation to this strategy'.

The overall strategy focuses on crime, young people and public health and is operationalized through strategies such as vigorous law enforcement, accessible treatment and a strong new emphasis on education and prevention. It is stated that 'multi-agency co-ordination, both at national and local levels will be required in order to make systematic progress towards these aims'. Addiction nurses have a clear role in achieving these aims, by contributing to better services for the following.

- Young people, especially in preventative, health promotion, harm-minimization and educational work and through collaboration with school based educational and health programmes. Drug prevention teams are set up in each health region to facilitate preventative action.
- Public health: by discouraging the misuse of drugs and encouraging the cessation of drug use through the provision of advice, counselling, family work, treatment and rehabilitation services. This may be put into practice through liaison with existing services, for example by working more closely with social workers, probation workers, health visitors, district nurses ,voluntary agencies. etc.

The Mental Health Nursing Review Team produced a report entitled *Working in Partnership: a Collaborative Approach to Care*, (Department of Health,1994). Clearly, the title of this report indicates a thrust to enhance collaborative practice and places emphasis on mental health nurses taking a central role in the provision of health services, including services for substance misuse. The report calls for greater links to be forged between mental health nurses working in substance misuse and services for mentally disordered offenders and the criminal justice system.

This recommendation urges not only stronger interprofessional links, but also better 'intraprofessional' links. It also serves as a reminder that particular subgroups of nursing specialty can become segregated from general nursing, creating communication barriers not dissimilar to those that exist between the different healthcare professions.

COLLABORATION IN EDUCATION AND TRAINING

The establishment of better interprofessional training opportunities may serve to explode the myths and misconceptions that individual professions hold about one another by increasing familiarity and dismantling barriers and boundaries. In 1995, The ENB for Nursing Midwifery and Health Visiting published a report entitled *Meeting the Education and Training Needs of Nurses, Midwives and Health Visitors in the Field of Substance Misuse* (ENB, 1995). As well as highlighting a range of general deficits in current substance misuse training programmes for nurses, the report also notes the current lack of multiprofessional education and training programmes. Training initiatives that are designed to be run on an interprofessional basis are more likely to foster effective interprofessional practice than those geared for a single profession. Rassool and Oyefeso (1993) have argued for a similar movement towards the development of more interprofessional training programmes.

The argument for interprofessional collaboration

Professional workers in substance misuse have been confronted with the challenge of adapting to a mode of interprofessional practice perhaps more than others. This is largely because substance misuse problems span the whole spectrum of health problems. These include sexual and mental health to child health, and from individual healthcare and communicable diseases to public health matters – with no major health field being an exception. Given the range of problems and health concerns encountered in the substance misuse field, it is argued that interprofessional collaboration is essential for effective practice. All substance misuse health-related problems which occur at the individual level, inevitably have an impact on public health although undoubtedly individual and public health strategies are distinctive.

Moores (1996) asserts that: 'Nurses who work in the area of substance misuse have a liaison and educational role which includes working with primary healthcare teams and staff in community services. This is an important aspect of their work as there are many varied and complex underlying issues, which frequently come to the fore when caring for people who misuse substances.' Addiction nurses often have to deal with complex issues: for example, the health, social and legal issues related to a pregnant substance misuser and her unborn child, or to a heavy drinker experiencing physical and emotional, economic and family difficulties. It is often the process of managing 'these varied and complex underlying issues' that necessitate that good interprofessional links are forged, if positive health outcomes are to be achieved. Such links may occur at local, regional, national or international level.

International collaboration

Substance misuse constitutes such a growing major global problem that there are good reasons for links being forged between countries and even continents, since experience can be shared and eventually policies and strategies could become more standardized. Improved collaboration between countries and cultures is an important facet of tackling drugs misuse globally. In the late 1980s The European Collaborating Centres in Addiction (ECCAS) was established to enhance the development of European drug research. Clancy (1995) states that 'the aim of this organization is to establish and develop sound and practical understanding of the impact of substance misuse on the individual, the family, the wider community and the best approaches and methods in dealing with it through a cohesive network of professionals across Europe'.

These aims are implemented through a variety of methods, such as educational and practice strategies, research and evaluation, supportive schemes and a commitment to forge further links with other similar organizations in an integrated and co-ordinated manner. The emphasis is on the membership of organizations and institutions rather than on individual membership, thus facilitating a team approach and preventing personal or idiosyncratic interests detracting from more general objectives. ECCAS has so far been very successful in achieving its overall aim, and should hopefully provide a positive model for other international collaborative initiatives. If international barriers and differences (for example language and cultural differences) could be minimized, the conflicts and challenges posed at a more local level (for example professional language/terminology differences and attitudes) could also be addressed successfully .

Conflicts and challenges

There are other problems and conflicts that impede successful interprofessional collaboration. For example, the establishment of an internal market environment within the health service, has led to the distinction between purchasers and providers of services. As purchasers are able to buy from several different providers, this encourages competition between providers. Consequently each provider strives to be more efficient and to offer a better quality service at the lowest possible cost. This situation could encourage professionals within each individual provider unit to become more territorial and less likely to share information with other providers. While such competitiveness is more likely to manifest among managerial personnel, it may also have some impact on clinical staff, who may face financial dilemmas about treatment options and interventions.

Nurses being the largest professional group within the substance misuse field arguably face more opportunities and challenges related to interprofessional practice than others. Traditionally, nurses have often been perceived as less prestigious and less influential than other groups such as doctors, despite the fact that they may be skilled and knowledgeable in their specialty. Of course this discrepancy is not peculiar to the substance misuse field, and the move towards interprofessional working may assist in establishing a more equitable status and lead to more power sharing as the individual professional groups develop more trusting relationships, based on improved knowledge and more positive and accurate perceptions of each other.

Kingdon (1992) indicates that interprofessional problems are not new but that 'philosophical and practical differences have bedevilled interprofessional collaboration'. Kingdon clarifies this point by citing the example of the philosophical differences between the 'medical model' of psychiatrists and the 'antipsychiatry' philosophy of social workers. While these two extreme positions have become the stereotype of the medical and social models of health (substance misuse nurses probably align themselves more closely with the social model), in reality few professionals are quite as polarized in their outlook. Nevertheless, these stereotypes are likely to act as a barrier to interprofessionalism, as such polarized perceptions tend to alienate one professional group from another, and diminish any conviction that a common understanding or collaboration is achievable. While this perspective suggests that doctors, nurses and social workers may experience problems in establishing true collaborative practice, it also suggests that groups such as social workers, probation workers, voluntary agencies may experience fewer problems in collaborating.

There is a prevalence of contradictory attitudes and opinions between the various professional factions, relating to complex areas of substance use. These areas include the legalization of currently illicit drugs, safe levels of alcohol consumption, law enforcement to combat illegal drug use/availability or the development of a more socially orientated strategy to the problem, and these conflicts of views only serve to perpetuate interprofessional rifts. These contradictory opinions represent differences in fundamental beliefs, attitudes and values. To some extent they are unavoidable as they are driven not only by factual knowledge, but are heavily influenced by cultural, religious and social factors. Nonetheless, more agreement may eventually be possible through better education and information being provided at all levels. Despite the existing problems, there is considerable cause for optimism that doctors, nurses and others working within the substance misuse field can move increasingly towards better collaboration, as exists already in many specialized fields where successful co-operative practice is commonplace. For example the close co-operation between substance misuse nurses, psychiatrists, midwives, obstetricians and social workers in managing the pregnant drug user. Reports from authors, such as Riley (1987), Green and Gossop (1988), Siney (1992), Dawe et al. (1992), provide evidence of successful interprofessional collaboration in this particular area of practice. Community Alcohol Teams (CATs) established in some areas have also been successful in establishing good collaborative links with GPs and other primary healthcare staff.

The success of such collaborative ventures appears to be based on establishing a facilitative ethos. Saunders *et al* (1995) describe a collaborative venture in the South Thames region, where addiction prevention counsellors (people with a health or social work professional backgrounds who are experienced or trained in addiction counselling) work closely with GPs. They describe the programmes: 'using a horizontal approach in sharing expertise. The counsellor is viewed as a peer and this has proved more acceptable than formal instruction from someone viewed as superior'. Undoubtedly, in most circumstances nurses, counsellors and social care staff are unlikely to be perceived as 'superior', but the horizontal approach described is a way of establishing an equitable, non-threatening relationship which is conducive to acceptance and effective communication, although there is a strong prerequisite that the counsellors are confident in their skills, knowledge and role. This can only be properly achieved through adequate educational and training provision, resulting in the development of a robust professional identity and role confidence.

CONCLUSION

Interprofessional collaboration is undoubtedly difficult to achieve, but this is not surprising given the complexities of service provision within the health field, and particularly in the substance misuse field. There is evidence that it can be achieved (Huxley, 1988; Stein and Test, 1980) and lead to improved health outcomes, indicating that existing barriers are well worth challenging. This review, has explored the concept of interprofessionalism from a theoretical, practical, policy and international perspective. The only way forward is to strive towards better interprofessional relations. In order to facilitate the transition towards collaboration, nurses need to make the best use of examples of successful collaborative ventures that are already available to them. Nursing led research that advances our knowledge and understanding about collaboration is to be encouraged and welcomed. There can be little doubt, in the light of present knowledge that there is an urgent and growing need for greater availability and access to training and education which is interdisciplinary in nature, at basic, intermediate and advanced levels.

The present climate should be welcomed by substance misuse nurses as an opportunity to change and improve both their practice and professional standing. Active contribution to public debate and participation in interprofessional conferences and publications provide opportunities for nursing to have a positive impact on future developments. Interprofessional practice is no longer optional, it is essential.

REFERENCES

Cartlidge, A.M. (1987) *Collaboration: A comparative study among primary healthcare professionals in four London Health authorities and Sixteen non-London Health Authorities*, University of Newcastle-Upon-Tyne.

Clancy, C. (1995) ECCAS's Annual Assembly. *Substance Misuse Bulletin*, **8**(2), 6–7.

Dawe, S., Gerada, C. and Strang, J. (1992) Establishment of a Liaison Service for Pregnant Opiate Users. *British Journal of Addiction*, **87**(6), 867–71.

Department of Health (1992) *The Health of the Nation: A Strategy for Health in England*, HMSO, London.

Department of Health (1994) *Working in Partnership: A Collaborative Approach to Care. Mental Health Nursing Review Team (MHNRT)*, HMSO, London.

English National Board for Nursing, Midwifery and Health Visiting (1995) *Meeting the Education and Training Needs of Nurses, Midwives and Health Visitors in the field of Substance Misuse*, ENB, London.

Ghodse, A.H. (1995) A Partnership in Research and Development. *Substance Misuse Bulletin*, **8**(1), 3.

Green, L. and Gossop, M. (1988) The Management of Pregnancy in Opiate Users. *Journal of Reproduction and Infant Psychology*, **6**(1), 51–7.

Huxley, P. (1988) *Social Work Practice in Mental Health: Teamwork*, Gower, Aldershot.

Kingdon, D.G. (1992) Interprofessional Collaboration in Mental Health. *Journal of Interprofessional Care*, **6**(2), 141–47.

Moores, Y. (1996) Letter. *Journal of Substance Misuse*, **1**(1),1.

Rassool, G.H. and Oyefeso, A.O. (1993) The Need for Substance Misuse Education in Health Studies Curriculum: A Case for Nursing Education. *Nurse Education Today*, **13**(2), 107–10.

Riley, D. (1987) The Management of The Pregnant Addict. *Bulletin of the Royal College of Psychiatrists*, **11**(11), 362–4.

Saunders, V., McShane, L. and Priestly, J. (1995) Addiction Prevention in Primary Care. *Substance Misuse Bulletin*, **8**(2), 8.

Siney, C. (1992) Great Expectations. *Nursing Standard*, **7**(8), 24–7.

Smoyak, S.A. (1977) Issues in Primary Care: Problems in interprofessional relations. *Bulletin of the New York Academy of Medicine*, **53**(1), 51–9.

Stein, L. and Test, M. (1980) Alternatives to mental health hospitals: Conceptual model treatment program and clinical evaluation. *Archives of General Psychiatry*, **37**, 392–97.

Tackling Drugs Together: A Strategy For England 1995–1998 (1995), HMSO, London.

PART FIVE

Service development and management

Needs assessment and policy development

21

Fiona Marshall

INTRODUCTION

The purpose of the NHS according to the Ministry of Health, in 1946, was to improve the physical and mental health of the nation. At its inception there was no real consideration of efficiency and effectiveness. Klein (1989) explained this in terms of the original expectations concerning the NHS; that demand would tail off after the pent up need had been satiated and that the NHS would eventually become self financing. However, these expectations were not realized, costs continued to spiral and, as the populations' expectations concerning health and well-being increased, together with paralleled increases in technology and medical innovations, demand spiralled. The NHS has been reorganized structurally many times since it was introduced.

In the 1980s the Griffiths Report (DHSS, 1983) introduced general management principles to the NHS, the former consensus management principles were swept aside, with themes of cost and quality taking on increasing importance. The NHS and Community Care Act (1990) has further expanded these themes by introducing the purchaser and provider model, with purchasers defining the quality and costs of care. Recently, the NHS executive (1995) described the purpose of the NHS: 'to secure through the resources available, the greatest possible improvement to the health of the people of England' (EL(95)105). The method advocated to achieve this goal is to arrive at decisions, using appropriate evidence about clinical effectiveness, thereby improving the clinical and cost effectiveness of services. These changes concerning quality are thought to be useful, and anecdotally treatment service staff are becoming more questioning in their approach. Practitioners have passed through a cultural shift, rather than taking a somewhat paternalistic approach. They have shifted to a rather more scientific approach and are thinking about outcomes of care and the processes involved in obtaining optimum outcomes. Generally, there is more health-related research which is aimed at comparing approaches and that uses control groups rather than uncontrolled and descriptive outcome studies. This scientific approach is still balanced by the art of care, staff experience and intuition. It would be a shame if the more human and individualistic approaches are forgotten during this time of rigorous testing and cost conscious approaches. These changes have obviously been influenced by many factors: people, generally have become more medically knowledgeable, advocacy and the patient-rights movements have had significant impacts and general information and communication channels are more effective, leading to more knowledge being shared.

The field of substance misuse in the UK has mirrored these changes. The field is somewhat complicated in that there are often many agencies involved. The subject can be an emotive one and there is some stigma attached to dependencies generally. There is a public health perspective, and the legal and forensic aspects can add a further dimension not common in other areas of healthcare.

In this chapter some of the recent policy developments that have affected substance misuse services are examined. Needs assessment in relation to substance misuse will then be examined with some examples of work carried out in relation to substance misuse. The particular issues concerning the purchaser–provider environment, service goals, outcomes, quality assurance and audit are also discussed. The chapter ends with a brief discussion on the nursing implications of all these areas of change.

APROACHES TO SUBSTANCE MISUSE

The 'British approach' to drug misuse

During the twentieth century the main focus on policy has been the treatment and rehabilitation of drug misusers and on prevention. The government advisory body, ACMD, has focused mainly on these areas. Since the mid 1980s HIV has added a further dimension to this treatment centred approach. Britain has traditionally placed drug misuse in the medical rather than enforcement domain. This approach has been coined as the 'British approach'. A more penal approach has been adopted in America and many European countries, with doctors having more limited powers to prescribe. There are, however, some significant initiatives such as the NHS and Community Care Act (1990), *Tackling Drugs Together* (1995) and the Health of the Nation (Department of Health, 1992) which need examination in the context of the new NHS and community care.

Tackling drug misuse 1986 and 1995

Since the mid 1980s there has been a significant shift in approach and the law enforcement angle has been given more prominence. The government's strategy Tackling Drug Misuse: a summary of the government's strategy, issued by the Home Office in 1985 and in 1986, began this process (Home Office, 1985; 1986). This strategy was the government's main approach through the late 1980s and early 1990s, the law enforcement angle becoming more important, with the Drug Trafficking Offences Act and others setting up higher penalties for trading in drugs. Stimpson (1987) described the 'war on drugs' and the economic model was highlighted, with the popular image of the evil drug pusher and the victim becoming more prominent. The later ACMD reports on HIV and drugs brought in a more sociomedical approach.

Tackling drugs together (1995)

The White Paper *Tackling Drugs Together* (1995) set a new national agenda, with three main areas of objectives;

- increasing the safety of communities from drug related crime;
- reducing the acceptability and availability of drugs to young people;
- reducing the health risks and other damage related to drug misuse.

This strategy is different from the 1986 government strategy, which was only issued by one government department. This new approach has been signed up to by many different government departments and is co-ordinated by one unit, Central Drugs Co-ordinating Unit.

The White Paper sets the nation's agenda for drug misuse with objectives on education, the penal service, the police, customs, and the health and local authorities. In the health/social field, it recommends the setting up of local drug action teams (DATs), by health authorities, with very senior, multi agency membership to oversee needs assessment and devise local performance indicators and strategies. Drug reference groups (DRGs) will inform this work and help to implement the decisions made by the DATs. Progress will be reported to the Central Drugs Co-ordinating Unit which, in turn, develops a picture of activity on all the action points of the national strategy. It is widely regretted that alcohol was not included in the new strategy, since much of the more local work will probably include alcohol.

HEALTH CIRCULARS

Since the 1980s, and Health Service Development Services for Drug Misusers HC(86)3 (DHSS, 1986), there have been many health and local authority circulars on the subject of drug misuse, HIV etc. The latest circular, HSG(95)26 (NHS Executive, 1995), covered the following areas; structured oral methadone maintenance programmes, outreach, the promotion of safer sexual practices, the role of GPs and training for them and others, HIV testing, wider health issues including hepatitis B and tuberculosis, the provision of drug services and prison issues.

THE HEALTH OF THE NATION

The White Paper *The Health of the Nation* (Department of Health, 1992) is a strategy aimed at improving health by setting targets for improvement in five main areas:

- cancers;
- coronary heart disease and strokes;
- accidents;
- HIV and AIDS;
- mental illness.

There is a specific target on reducing alcohol consumption, and alcohol is mentioned in all of the main areas. For drug misuse the target involves reducing injecting behaviour.

THE NHS AND COMMUNITY CARE ACT (1990)

This Act carried on two of the main health and social care themes of the 1980s; the introduction of general management principles into the NHS, controlling where funds go and for what service and to further care in the community. At the time of the Act's introduction, the selling point was that there was patient choice and resources would follow the patient. In practice this has not really happened as health authorities have drawn up many block contracts with local providers so it is difficult for patients to specify choice and only in exceptional cases are extra-contractual referrals made. Health authorities are expected to assess the health needs of their resident populations, and commission appropriate healthcare responses.

Local authorities were allocated money to purchase packages of social care, based on individual need. The assessment of need was supposed to be separated from the budget management with case managers purchasing the care to satisfy the identified need. This process is now means tested, and people who are deemed able, have to contribute to the costs. Originally money for drug and alcohol social care (mainly rehabilitation) was to be ring fenced, as there were fears that the needs of this group would be missed when considering the social care needs of children, the elderly and the disabled. The ring fencing did not happen. In practice the drugs and alcohol non statutory agencies appear to have coped very well with having to chase funding for clients from many different local authorities. However, it is still very early days after such significant changes, and time will tell.

NEEDS ASSESSMENT

One of the major changes initiated by the NHS and Community Care Act (1990) was the commissioning of services, the health authorities were charged with assessing the healthcare needs of the catchment area population, developing strategies to address those needs and then purchasing appropriate services. The application of market principles, defining what is being purchased and costing activity, purchasing according to price, quality and acceptability, defining what will be spent on what sounds fairly easy until the complexity of all healthcare systems and their interdependency is considered.

The introduction of the cultural shift to supplying healthcare according to assessed need has been interesting. Commissioners of services have been given the responsibility of defining need and developing appropriate healthcare responses. In some areas of healthcare this appears relatively simple, the numbers of, say, hip replacements needed for a given population could be assessed by examining previous years' activity. This sort of information was fairly easily accessed and covered many years. However, even less contentious areas of healthcare such as hip replacements can arouse major local outrage when people have to wait long periods for their operations, questions around rationing, poor management of resources and other such issues are quickly aired.

Drug and alcohol needs assessment.

In the drugs and alcohol field the question of needs assessment is much more complex when viewed as a health or social need. Substance misusers are not an homogenous group with homogenous required responses.

Needs assessment and alcohol

Edwards and Unnithal (1994), when considering alcohol, described using information from the general household surveys (GHS) to consider the prevalence of hazardous drinking. They also categorized drinkers into three main categories:

- category I: excessive drinking without occurrence of problems or dependence;
- category II: excessive drinking with occurrence of problems but without established dependence;
- category III: excessive drinking with problems and dependence.

Edwards and Unnithal (1994) advocated that the GHS data could then be applied to this categorization and that some indication of need could be signalled. Certainly local household surveys could be carried out at intervals to assess trends in need for services. Additional indicators can be used such as the hospital patient administration systems, Korner data, specialist service utilization, liver cirrhosis incidence, accident and emergency data, drink driving offences, drunk and disorderly offences and probation figures can be used to generate a picture of need and a view on trends. The South Thames (West) Regional Substance Use database (SUD) also records alcohol as a substance of misuse and demographic information. The SUD can therefore be used as an additional source of information on alcohol problems. One health authority also worked closely with the local Licensed Victuallers Association which monitors the amounts of alcohol sold in an area over a period and then calculate per capita consumption.

Needs assessment and drug misuse

Prevalence studies

Local prevalence studies can be conducted to estimate the incidence of drug misuse in specified areas (Hartnoll *et al.*, 1985; Pattison *et al.*, 1982). Most prevalence studies utilize methods devised in the field of sociology and ethnography such as 'snowballing' where people in contact with services are asked to nominate people they know. These are in turn contacted until the 'tracks' dry up. Such techniques enable the researchers to contact people not previously in contact with services and provide a picture of unmet need. This is also an effective approach in obtaining user involvement in shaping services and service commissioning. All such studies indicate that the level of problematic drug use is five, seven or ten times the rate indicated in the Home Office Addicts Index. Most of these studies have been carried out in urban areas and developing a picture of need in rural areas may require more elaborate methodologies.

Home Office Index and the regional databases

Needs assessments traditionally consider data which is already available such as the Home Office Addicts Index. All doctors are statutorily required to notify any patient they know or suspect to be addicted to the class A drugs to the Addicts Index. This Index is known to be under utilized and the figures published are an underestimate of the drug using population. In 1989, the Department of Health required each region in the country to set up regional drugs databases, with agencies dealing with drug users requested to report new episodes or contacts to the databases, providing information on the drugs used and some demographic information. The purpose of the databases was to enhance the level of information on trends concerning drug use. General practitioners and agencies, such as social services and probation as well as accident and emergency departments, are also expected to contribute to the databases. At present most contributors to the databases are still specialist drug agencies. Most databases have been in operation for some four or five years and some valuable information is now being generated. They were never intended to provide hard figures on numbers of addicts, or service activity as only new contacts are recorded, but information on trends can be useful when planning healthcare.

Other data

Police data can also be useful when trying to develop a picture of need. The numbers of arrests and cautions can indicate levels of drug-related activity, but can be influenced by changes in police strategies and priorities over time. The customs and excise figures on seizures can also indicate levels of drug-related activity, but these figures are subject to 'blips' when large hauls are made and are often not directly relevant to health authorities. Information on the street price of drugs and their purity can also indicate availability and subsequent potential healthcare needs.

Figures on the number of accidental overdoses, accidents involving intoxication, complications of injecting etc. can be gleaned from accident and emergency departments. Mortality figures and other indicators such as hepatitis C incidence can also be used over time to assess the extent of healthcare needs and the potential costs to services.

Organizing needs assessments

Strang (1994) when considering needs assessment for problem drug misuse, described falling under physical, psychological and/ or social headings. He suggested there are seven target groups whose needs should be considered when assessing healthcare need:

- the dependent user – those who could experience classical withdrawal syndrome;
- the injector – those needing attention in terms of reducing the incidence of septicaemia, HIV hepatitis B and C;
- the intoxicated drug user – this is a transitory phase, but individuals may need care to protect their wellbeing;
- the user in withdrawal – these individuals may need specific emergency care especially those withdrawing from barbiturates, benzodiazepines as these states can be life-threatening, withdrawing opiate users also need attention;
- drug user co-morbidity – drug users who have additional drug associated complications such as subacute bacterial endocarditis, HIV related illness, hepatitis B and C;
- the individual at risk (tomorrow's patient);
- the addict in recovery;
- the pregnant addict – this category was suggested to be a further subcategory in that pregnant drug users require additional consideration.

It could be argued that this framework may be a useful one to use when assessing health need in a population. However, it could also be argued that these seven categories are rather physically defined and the needs of people not using opiates or those experiencing mainly psychological and social problems are not easily addressed in this model. The counselling and advice needs of families and carers are definitely not considered in this model.

It may be better to organize a needs assessment using a prevention model; considering health needs from primary, secondary and tertiary perspectives. This could help in developing strategies and therefore services/ responses targeted at different levels of need. This approach could then be more responsive, aiming responses at different needs, rather than at specific substances misused. The primary level of need would cover the areas concerning why people use in the first instance and at reducing harm. The secondary level would involve the active treatment, intervention and harm reduction of the misusers and their carers and the general population. Finally, the tertiary level would consider those chronic users who have experienced physical harm and who need some level of rehabilitation/ recovery.

This type of approach would facilitate the assessment of need of the group at the early stage of drug use (often called recreational or occasional users) who may be in need of the specialist treatment services in the future. Needs assessment of a population developed in this way could be more dynamic, and represent a more accurate, preventative picture, rather than a fatalistic, often self-fulfilling prophecy which demands yet more acute tertiary level services and responses. It would also be easier to develop more effective early intervention services such as peer education programmes, counselling, work/ skills based projects alongside the very necessary active treatment services.

None of these indicators are therefore useful on their own, rather a composite picture needs to be developed. The transient nature of drug users, the frequently illicit nature of drug misuse, the nature of addiction and the fact that 'recreational'/occasional drug users have healthcare needs make the picture even more complex. It is much better to assess need over a period, examining trends and patterns when considering developing purchaser strategies. Obviously the two areas of work should occur in tandem, informing each other in a dynamic process. The DATs and DRGs, with multi agency membership, have a significant role to play in this, developing a proactive, rather than reactive approach, but this is a difficult balancing act. There are always political and emotive issues to consider in the healthcare arena, episodes such as ecstasy related deaths, the problem of inappropriately discarded injecting equipment and stigma/ prejudice will always need to be considered.

RANGE OF SERVICES TO BE CONSIDERED

When conducting a full needs assessment the services available also need to be considered. There are a range of services which are necessary:

- advice and information;
- counselling;
- needle exchange;
- prescribing – rapid detoxification,

- long term prescribing,
- slow detoxification,
- symptom control (in terms of cocaine, amphetamines, etc.);
- aftercare/ rehabilitation;
- family/ carer support;
- crisis intervention;
- prevention/ early intervention;
- services geared to particular groups such as young people, women, pregnant users, ethnic minorities, the homeless;
- general medical/ healthcare.

Not all these services should be funded with health funds as there is always an element of social care and probation/prison services which need to be involved in this. Also not all these services need to be drug or alcohol specialists, some services such as those for young people are better provided in a generalist setting. It is not always useful to develop separate services for substance misusers. A full needs assessment, therefore, will need to take account of all services, general and specialist in order to complete the process arriving at decisions concerning the appropriate healthcare response.

PURCHASER AND PROVIDER ISSUES

The illegal drugs scene is a market in itself, commodities are bought and sold. Alcohol is always available from a variety of outlets. Drug users and to a lesser extent alcohol users have been known to shop around for services and prescribed drugs with a market value. Health commissioners have a responsibility to improve the health of their resident population and wider public health issues rather than individual cases. Commissioners have to balance the health needs of different groups and are guided by the NHS executive and the effectiveness and costs are becoming ever more important. They also have to agree priorities with local authorities. Purchasers of healthcare may also be influenced by competing providers, offering similar sounding services at markedly lower prices.

Providers of services are in direct contact with service users and may develop different perspectives on priorities. Teams can also develop 'passions' for certain projects which may not be within the commissioners set of priorities. New initiatives, while having a clear clinical benefit for certain groups may not have an obvious impact when considering the whole.

These general factors are also complicated by the fact that prescriptions of drugs are attractive to drug misusers. Also changes in behaviour for all of us is difficult, be it giving up smoking, taking up regular exercise, stopping or controlling drinking or modifying drugtaking behaviour. Drug and to a lesser extent alcohol services could attract more clients by introducing liberal prescribing practices. This practice could have limited health benefits, and in some circumstances be positively dangerous, but could attract additional funding. This situation is also complicated by the fact that there are often many different providers, statutory, non-statutory and voluntary in most localities. Commissioners need to develop quite sophisticated monitoring and quality control mechanisms. The internal market model does not therefore marry well with the substance misuse services.

Contracting processes

Contracting is usually conducted in an annual cycle. At present, health commissioners produce draft purchasing intentions in September for the following financial year. These documents are overall statements of the authority's plans, indicating the general approach in each area. They are then circulated for comment, and there are usually public meetings to discuss the plans. The final purchasing intentions are published in the December after having been discussed with the NHS executive regional office. The more detailed contracting arrangements are finalized in the January, February and March for the forthcoming year.

Types of contracts

There are three main types of contracts; block, cost-volume and cost per case contracts.

Block contract
The block contract is the most basic form of contract, the purchaser pays an agreed sum of money for access to a range of services. This has disadvantages and advantages in that the provider has to continue providing services even if there is increased demand involving additional costs, but there is a guaranteed sum of money. The purchaser does not have to be provided with detailed information, but does know that the services for its residents will be provided.

Cost-volume contract
The cost-volume contract defines a given level of activity for an agreed sum. If activity exceeds the given levels of activity, an additional sum is paid for further activity, a maximum ceiling is usually agreed. Purchasers usually retain a contingency fund for these contracts and balance need in different areas when activity exceeds the original agreements.

Cost per case contract
The cost per case contract is less common and is rarely used in the mental health field where payment is made for individual cases. Providers do not usually use this form of contract as it entails a great deal of administration. In substance misuse these types of contracts may be used to fund the healthcare elements of an individuals' social care placement, usually if detoxification is needed, but there can be other packages which have a health aspect. For further reading see specialist works such as the York Health Economics Consortium (1993).

Service goals and treatment outcomes

One of the best strategies for providers dealing with a competitive funding environment is to have clear and widely agreed service goals and objectives. Commissioners have a significant role in helping services to define their goals and areas of activity. If communication is open, people will understand the processes involved and there is less room for controversy and competition. Services can then work together more constructively when the element of competition for funds is removed, patients and clients can be referred between services according to clinical need and which service can best address that need at that time.

The need for efficiency and cost effectiveness will still need to be continually addressed, but the process will be more constructive and clients will ultimately benefit from such an approach. Outcome measurement is an important and developing area. If the service goals are clearly stated outcomes are somewhat easier to define. In the field of addiction some would define a successful outcome as abstinence, however, as previously discussed, drug problems are usually considered to have physical, psychological and social dimensions. Edwards and Unnithal (1994), on considering the effectiveness and treatment of alcohol problems stated that the overriding conclusion is that 'different drinking problems require different types of treatment'. They also suggest that treatment needs to be matched to the individual patient and that the patient should be allowed to choose. If a pregnant, injecting HIV positive and homeless drug user approaches a service the ultimate goal of treatment may be abstinence. There could be many successful stages of treatment with differing goals ranging from persuading the patient to attend antenatal care, facilitating her finding accommodation, stabilizing her on oral methadone etc. Outcome measurement should be considered in terms of service goals, and could be assessed in terms of behaviour change against care plans.

Strang (1994) suggested it might be more useful to consider outcomes in terms of levels. The first level considering basic activity data, how many people were in contact with an agency, completely new cases, cases who had been in contact with the agency previously and the residual caseload. The second level of outcome measurement, Strang suggested, would involve recording how long people stayed in contact with the agency and considering how long between time of first use of a drug and contact with the agency, relapse rates, how long between relapse and recontacting the agency. The idea for this level is that successful agencies would have shorter periods of time between relapse and recontact. The author of this chapter feels this may not be a very useful approach because there are external factors which may affect the contact times such as increased police activity, a reduced availability of street drugs, concerns about adulterated drugs or increases in the price of drugs. There is also a danger that commissioners may compare different services in different areas, and conclusions about services could be inappropriately made. This measure could be used, however, to contribute to the picture of unmet need.

Ghodse (1987) advocates considering events occurring across the district:

- acute intoxication–overdoses seen in A and E departments, deaths linked to drugs;
- acute withdrawal–numbers of acute cases seen by GPs, A and E departments, hospital admissions linked with acute withdrawal;
- dependence–numbers of people seen in the specialist services, neonatal withdrawals;
- physical complications linked with drug misuse;
- psychiatric conditions linked with drug misuse;
- social problems linked with drug misuse.

The problem with such an approach is that such measurements could be expensive in terms of manpower, even in these days of computerization such details are rarely routinely recorded. Also, should such an exercise be carried out it could only indicate the outcomes of the whole portfolio of services and not individual agencies teams. However, such an exercise would inform the whole needs assessment process very well and could form part of a cycle of needs assessment ascertaining effective commissioning.

Quality assurance and audit

Quality assurance and audit are usually internal activities of teams or organizations, but it is useful to share the results of these activities with purchasers. Outcome measurement is a form of quality measurement. Services can devise their own methods of measuring outcomes, individual care plans can be used, progress should be assessed against these plans. and a simple system of recording the results can be devised. As with all such exercises the more methodical the process the clearer the picture developed. Ryder (1993) stated that it is currently difficult to define the effects that current healthcare provision has on health outcomes and many clinicians and academics are still battling with the issue. However, he does not think this is a good enough reason not to continue trying! Medical and nursing audit may be approached by examining simple processes such as waiting lists, management, admission rates, and duration of treatment.

Quality can also be measured in terms of structure, for example, what the buildings and accommodation look like, staff appearance, notices, or whether clients/patients are aware of the complaints procedure. The process of care is also a quality indicator, nursing and medical audit tend to concentrate on this area with varying degrees of success. These include issues such as those concerning staff communication, how sensitive the staff are to differing groups of patients, how long people have to wait for a first assessment appointment, and whether appointment times are kept.

Patients' satisfaction is also an indicator of quality. In the field of substance misuse, as with most of the other areas, there are the dimensions influenced by the fact that service users are often ambivalent about change, and may feel that they, for example, would like higher doses of the prescribed drugs, would like injectable drugs etc. However, there are areas which could be examined effectively.

- Do you understand your care programme?
- Are you seen at the time of your appointment?
- Do you feel you have enough time to discuss problems?
- Do you know how to complain about anything?
- Do you feel your care is confidential to the team?

Nursing implications

Nurses are all too often ignorant about the new arrangements, viewing all the contracting arrangements as 'management's' role and nothing to do with them. There are many things addiction nurses can and should be involved in, from educating commissioners about the service, devising new and innovative ways of measuring quality and auditing processes of care to liaising with other services (NHS Executive, 1994). There is a growing importance in defining expected service goals and outcomes.

Addiction nurses have a vital role to play in this whole area, from contributing to writing policies, mission statements and service philosophies and to ensure these policies are enacted and updated as appropriate. Improving communication with patients/ clients, managers, purchasers, other service providers are also very much the nurses' role. To carry out these tasks it is also important for nurses to remain up to date and eclectic in their thinking. It is not useful nowadays to read only the specialist and clinical journals, we all need to be more politically (with a small 'p' and a large 'P') aware in order to keep abreast of all developments.

CONCLUSION

The implications of the health service changes introduced at the beginning of the 1990s are only really beginning to have an effect in the mid 1990s. Some services have already become casualties of the internal market, despite it being acknowledged that needs assessment is in its infancy. Commissioning is an art and not a science and there is no common agreement on what is an effective service, and what outcomes should be measured.

The split between purchasers and providers is widening. There is a danger that the split can become too wide, with communication between providers and purchasers becoming too caught up in costs, volumes and activity and not about the real issues. Providers could become competitive, with some becoming casualties of the processes. Substance misuse is an endemic problem, there are plenty of people in need of assistance, many not using the already busy services. Many different services are needed, it is hoped that sensitive needs assessment can develop effective responses all aimed at reducing harm or at least minimizing harm to the individual and the general population.

REFERENCES

Department of Health (1992) *The Health of the Nation: a strategy for England*, HMSO, London.

Department of Health and Social Security (1983) *NHS Management Enquiry (The Griffiths Report) DA(83)38*, DHSS, London.

Department of Health and Social Security (1986) *Health Service Development Services for Drug Misusers HC(86)3 and LAC(86)5*, DHSS, London.

Edwards, G. and Unnithal, S. (1994) Alcohol Misuse, in *Health Care Needs Assessment, Vol. 2* (eds A. Stevens and J. Raftery), Radcliffe Medical Press, Oxford.

Ghodse, A.H. (1987) Indicators of the extent of drug-related health problems, in *Psychoactive drugs and health problems* (eds J. Idanpaan-Heikkila, A.H. Ghodse and I. Khan), World Health Organisation, Geneva.

Hartnoll, R.L., Lewis, R., Micheson, M. and Bryer, S. (1985) Estimating the prevalence of opiod dependence. *Lancet*, **1**(8422), 203–5.

Home Office (1985) *Tackling Drug Misuse: a summary of the government's strategy*, 1st edn, HMSO, London.

Home Office (1986) *Tackling Drug Misuse: a summary of the government's strategy*, 2nd edn, HMSO, London.

Klein, R. (1989) *The politics of the National Health Service*, 2nd ed, Longman, London.

NHS Executive (1994) *Building a stronger team: the nursing contribution to purchasing*, HMSO, London.

NHS Executive (1995) *Health authority drug misuse services 1995/6, HSG(95)26*, HMSO, London.

NHS Executive/Department of Health (1995) *Improving the effectiveness of clinical services EL(95)105*, HMSO, London.

Pattison, C.J., Barnes, E.A. and Thorely, A. (1982) *Tyneside drug prevalence and indicators study* (report to the Department of Health), Centre for Alcohol and Drugs Studies, Newcastle.

Ryder, S. (1993) Reviewing the work undertaken by the organization, in *Business Planning for providers of healthcare services*, York Health Economics Consortium, Longman, Harlow.

Stimpson, G. (1987) The war on heroin, in *A land fit for heroin?* (eds N. Dorn and N. South), MacMillan Education, Houndsmills.

Strang, J. (1994) *Drug Misuse, in Health Care Needs Assessment, Vol. 2* (eds A. Stevens and J. Raftery), Radcliffe Medical Press, Oxford.

Tackling Drugs Together (1995), HMSO, London.

York Health Economics Consortium (1993), *Business Planning for providers of healthcare services*, Longman, Harlow.

Community substance misuse team: management and practice

22

Alan Staff

INTRODUCTION

The development of a network of multidisciplinary community based drug teams in the 1980s, prompted largely through the ACMD *Treatment and Rehabilitation Report* (ACMD, 1982) and facilitated by central funding initiative, saw a sudden rush to establish specialist units with little previous research to draw upon. Strang and Clement (1994), in their commentary on the rise of the community drug team (CDT), note that the first team was established in 1983 and that by 1991 more than half of the 192 district health authorities in England had such a team. The overwhelming perception of this emerging community substance misuse team was one that varied in function and style according to the philosophical bias of the lead individual or organization (Strang and Clement, 1994). They evolved in a host of different forms, and were not always responsive to local requirements. In fact, today, it is still very difficult to define the quintessential community substance misuse team, and harder still to find any guidance on what this curious beast actually should be.

This chapter will address some of the most pressing issues facing addiction nurses, managers, planners and purchasers of substance misuse services. It does not attempt to be a definitive guide but specific areas have been chosen by the author as those most relevant to enhancing professional practice in today's purchaser/provider climate. In placing these issues in historical context, consideration is given to the changing nature of management as a response to socioeconomic and political factors.

AIMS OF SUBSTANCE MISUSE SERVICES

In the 1990s, a widely held view by community substance misuse teams was to attract and hold as many drug users as possible. This offer resulted in a clear failure to grasp the size of the problem, or the basic economics of providing what would in effect become a demand led service. So what should be the aims of a substance misuse service?

To advise or to prescribe?

Donmall *et al.* (1989) and Strang and Clement (1994) both discuss the early concept of a community drug team as a geographically limited service which would provide support and education to existing generic services. The multidisciplinary basis of the teams was designed to facilitate the formation of support and dialogue across all agencies. Significantly, however, the first community drug team accepted that there should be a role for the service to provide direct treatment facilities.

Clearly the original concept was for a consultative agency mobilizing generic services to work more effectively. This plan relied totally on the willingness of other agencies, particularly primary healthcare, to increase their level of input and, in some cases, to change their approach to the illegal drug using community. The reality of course was that there wasn't widespread eagerness to take on this role (Greenwood, 1992; Waller, 1993), leaving drug teams with a simple choice. Either they should continue to try to work with the minority of users presenting who either had existing support systems or did not require medical intervention, or seek to fill the gap themselves by becoming direct service providers, taking on a role broadly similar to that of the old DDU at a more local level. The effect of this has been well documented by Wilson (1992) with drug teams who had set out with the objective of reaching all drug misusers finding themselves focusing on male, white opiate users and being regarded by their client group as a methadone service.

Harm-minimization or treatment?

The emergence of HIV as a major issue in the 1980s triggered a change in focus for many agencies, not least because a considerable amount of funding was made available for providers to bid for under the guise of HIV prevention initiatives. Suddenly teams became funded mainly by HIV allocated money which dictated the way in which they operated and the aim shifted towards a public health model of harm-minimization. Services began to emerge whose whole philosophy it appeared was to create a comfortable and accepting environment for drug use, held to ransom almost by the threat that drug users may threaten society as we know it if they should be denied any service or be alienated in any way. As needle exchanges, mobile units, sex industry workers and drug prescribing centres blossomed in this initial euphoria (Staff, 1993), a confusion began to arise, largely between medical and social philosophies, about what were the most important aims, and the injecting drug user became the main focus of service attention.

Target setting and outcomes

By the mid 1990s, with the changes in contract culture, it has become vital that teams are able to express clearly what they are aiming to achieve, including targets and time frames. However, with the separation between purchaser and provider, there is perhaps no longer room for the provider led reactive responses of earlier years. With the establishment of the DAT and DRG, initiated by the White Paper *Tackling Drugs Together* (1995), purchasers are expected to be clear about the services they wish to buy and for what reason. This may have direct implication for whether drug and alcohol teams are seen as separate entities or should be provided within a single service/agency.

Power *et al.* (1991) anticipated this change by detailing an action research based model for deciding the activity of their service. This sets out the clear aim of reducing the spread of HIV among injecting drug users. It established a data collection and analysis system, and from this analysis drew up a service structure which concentrated its work on those aspects found to be most effective.

Such a detached approach might, in today's terminology, be seen as 'rationing' and would be anathema to many workers brought up on the collectivist ideal of responding to each and every demand, free at the point of delivery. Nevertheless, substance misuse teams must make a decision about whether they wish to be seen as offering effective interventions based on some form of research methodology, with all the uncomfortable issues around cost effectiveness and accountability, or whether they will continue to operate on the 'because it feels right' basis which may make the workers feel good but is unlikely to impress those with a responsibility to ensure that limited public funding is used most efficiently.

SERVICE PHILOSOPHY

There are two fundamental approaches which dominate the world of substance misuse and provide a constant intellectual battlefield for the protagonists on both sides. The first is the abstinence versus control debate which has entered an interesting phase combining with current market led ideology. Market philosophy demands that the state should take a minimal controlling role, with individuals deciding for themselves how they choose to care for themselves within their financial means. This could suggest complete abdication by the state of any substance misuse intervention thereby leaving supply and demand to find their own levels. However, there is little political likelihood of such a radical move, and this dichotomy has caused much strain among planners and service managers who may receive a somewhat confused message. The second major debate revolves around the discussion of whether in fact substance misuse should be approached from a medical or a psychosocial perspective.

Influential in the process of defining the role of a substance misuse team are factors such as the demographic nature of the area served, the philosophical model of the more senior personnel within the provider network, and the traditional mores of the existing service. For instance, an urban area may find it most effective to centralize services thereby maximizing resources, whereas a service operating in a predominantly rural community may find that the most effective means of reaching its population is through the use of outreach base models or satellite networks. Such a rational approach, however, may become influenced by historical siting of services in psychiatric units, based around consultants and a medicalized system. This may have the effect of encouraging the illness model, generally more prevalent in the alcohol field, or a reliance on pharmacological interventions. Some of the more innovative schemes in the country have arisen through the establishing of drug teams either within community units or under the umbrella of a non-statutory organization often as an attempt to break out of what is sometimes perceived as a medically dominated field. On the other hand, some teams have deliberately set out to avoid the direct service role and have adopted the role of advisory services without any medical input. This may force the service into an advocacy role which depends entirely on the ability of other services to pick up the medicalized aspects of care.

The majority of CDTs have attempted to provide as full a range of services as possible, including the employing of outreach workers, needle exchange workers, methadone clinic staff and as wide a range of disciplines and approaches as they can justify. The philosophy behind this states that drug users are traditionally poor users of other services and therefore the specialist services which do have the ability to attract drug users should take advantage of the 'window of opportunity.' They should seek to provide a menu of options to retain the client by finding something which the service can offer to improve their lives. The model which emerges from this is based less on treatment outcomes and more on improving the quality of life of the target group, thereby decreasing the negative effects of drug misuse. The provider using this model becomes a specialist service offering generic services to a specific client group. This feels good for the worker as the 'benevolent helper', and ensures that the client is able to access all the services needed. However, it also discourages the involvement of generic services and ensures the continuing alienation of drug misusing individuals who are encouraged to see themselves as a 'special' category of individuals.

Choice of model

Whichever model is adopted, it is vital that any professional service is aware of the dangers inherent in creating and maintaining a dependency culture among its clients through being seen as the only ones who can help. It is also apparent that agencies who model themselves on a single philosophical model are unlikely to offer services which meet all the needs or wishes of the whole drug misusing community, so the eclectic multidisciplinary approach remains the dominant model. For historical reasons, however, the achievement of such a rational balance is rare, with strong medical influences being the most common dominant factor. Managers who wish to ensure an eclectic approach are likely to spend considerable time balancing the demands of a range of influential professional groups.

This is less often the case in the non-statutory sector however, where a defined philosophical approach is often offered as a key selling point. Purchasers therefore must be clear about what they wish to purchase, and the agency must be clear about what it is able to do within the limitations of its resources and its orientation.

Contract culture

The fundamentally evolutionary nature of most teams, together with the difficulties that arose following the funding of many mainstream drug services from ring-fenced HIV finance, meant that when the time came for purchasers to grasp the nettle and seek to define the activity of a service for contracting purposes, they were faced with a seriously complex situation. Drug agencies in particular were operating a range of services from education and awareness through helplines, harm-minimization work, outreach, treatment, aftercare, carers' support, HIV testing, programmes for the criminal justice system and a host of locally devised and sometimes ill defined functions which in some cases were frankly made up as they went along.

Most still operated under the prime directive of attracting the maximum clients into the service without recognizing that within the new purchasing arrangements money did not follow the patient. It is apparent that many health authorities and DAT have made as their first priority the appointment of a co-ordinator to enable planning and purchasing. Given that the majority of services have ended up within Trusts however, one of the most important tasks facing substance misuse services today is to ensure that some form of contract is made which both acknowledges the range of activities required and sets reasonable levels of activity within that range. Types of contract are discussed in chapter 21.

When there are a range of providers an arrangement may be made for each agency to provide specified aspects of service within an overall strategy, frequently known as a service level agreement. Some agencies carry this further entering into partnership arrangements to provide joint care of which the three-way contract (for example between a non-statutory agency, a statutory agency and the health authority) is a type.

The most fundamental change for the substance misuse team is that the clinicians and specialists no longer define need and priority without challenge, the responsibility for needs assessment and provision of services is now with the purchaser. The service which operated largely in response to demand is now subject to a contract or contracts which are supposedly needs led, and must increasingly be more concerned about the quality and efficiency of what it is doing rather than worrying about what it is not doing.

Quality and standards

The introduction of audit has led to an increase in accountability for substance misuse services as a whole. This has brought into focus the need for the purchasers to know what they are buying, the staff to know exactly what they are supposed to be doing and, with the advent of the Patient's Charter, the public to know what they are getting. In order to standardize and clarify what the service does it is vital to produce standards and policies.

A policy sets out to state clearly what the response of the service is to a given situation, and it is the reference point for staff and public to define whether the service is operating within its operational norms. A policy may be imposed by a Trust or governing body, it may be required to comply with legislation or it may be locally devised. However, once agreed a policy becomes a binding document in law, breach of which may be seen as unprofessional conduct. Key policies for a service will include guidelines for working with under 16-year-olds, confidentiality, prescribing, HIV counselling and testing, referrals, record keeping and security, home visiting, advising about self-injection and many others. Each of the above deals with a situation where the rights of clients, staff and carers need to be made explicit.

A standard defines the minimum constituents of a given activity. For instance, the Patient's Charter states that clients should be dealt with by someone competent to carry out the procedure as well as requiring services to state the time-scale for a client to access this. A standard on assessment therefore should indicate the level of training required to perform this function as well as how long it took for the person to be seen. Many standards are displayed publicly and invite the public to complain if the standard is not met. It is important therefore to make a standard achievable, and Dufficy and Hager (1993) offer some helpful advice on this subject .

With things changing as rapidly as they are, it is sensible for policies, procedures and standards to be reviewed regularly to ensure they still meet their purpose. Many agencies have either internal or external audit systems which should base much of their work on the standards of an agency and to what extent that agency kept within those standards. It is therefore in the interests of the agency staff to ensure these standards are current and relevant. Often clinicians resent audit as an intrusion into their knowledge-base and professional integrity, but many staff are finding great reassurance in having their boundaries defined.

Cochrane (1989), in a discussion of role security for drug workers, and Wilson (1992), in examining role uncertainty and the importance of teamwork, both stress the requirement for all staff to understand their roles clearly and to be aware of the boundaries and their own value within a team. The development of clear operational policies is a first step towards clarifying individual roles and functions.

Skill mix

Clarification about the function of a service and the standards that are required makes for a more task-centred workstyle as opposed to the responsive instinctive model previously applied. When functions were blurred and every worker was an independent practitioner, it meant that often all the workers in a team had similar functions regardless of professional background under the ubiquitous title 'drug worker'. This created much unease among professional groups who felt de-skilled, and led to the often posed question why do you need a highly paid and qualified nurse/social worker etc. to do a job which in many non-statutory agencies is carried out equally well by non-qualified staff? A small rural service for example needs to equip each service member with as many skills as possible, because it is not possible to centralize the service and split areas of work in the same way as an urban service. However, it can utilize other community agency resources to augment its range of options. A centralized service is much more open to skill mix options, where individuals of different grades and backgrounds carry out separate expert functions.

Supervision

While supervision is covered elsewhere in this book (chapter 24), it remains an important management tool and deserves some mention here. Traditionally, nurses and other staff who have elected to work in substance misuse have been regarded as maverick and difficult to manage. The opportunity for independent autonomous working practices in a specialism where the client group is frequently operating in an illegal under-world or subculture is fraught with danger. Too frequently it leads to staff becoming over involved, over stressed or stretching the boundaries of professional conduct sometimes beyond a safe limit, albeit for laudable purposes.

The pressures on Trusts to reduce managerial overheads often leads to a reduction in direct managerial involvement in teams, and it is essential that staff have access to regular formal supervision. Often managers from health service backgrounds have little concept of the type of supervision with which social workers for instance are familiar, seeing instead a form of benevolent oversight as meeting the needs of staff. Unfortunately, some of the more experienced nursing staff tend to collude with this through adopting a detached macho stance of not requiring advice or help from anyone. The most common effect of this is burnout and dangerous practice, which may end in serious trouble at some stage (Spratley, 1991). An effective system of supervision combines managerial, peer and external models to ensure not only that practice is safe and effective, but also that the staff carrying it out are supported, valued and allowed space to consider their own activities in a reflective manner.

While some managers may consider such comprehensive supervision an expensive luxury, the effects of poor staff retention, sickness and litigation could be very much more so. Ovretveit (1992) holds that quality in healthcare has three components namely quality in service delivery to clients and carers, professional quality in carrying out activities in an acceptable manner and management quality which looks to the most efficient and productive use of resources. For any manager the staff available are the most potent, valuable but also potentially fragile resources they have and, as such, need to be looked after. For the individual staff member it should be remembered that everyone has an obligation to ensure that they are identifying their own needs to managers and essentially offering as much support as possible to each other.

CONCLUSION

In whatever way a service is established and run, it is still expected to evaluate its effectiveness and thereby justify its existence. Gillam *et al.* (1992) suggest frameworks for evaluation but recognize that much depends on just what is considered to denote success. After all, how easy would it be to set up any sort of control group? Curson (1991) pointed out that treatment efficacy is not the single most important question. However, it offers a valuable start to the debate and quotes Griffith Edwards' maxim that treatment is '… at best a timely nudge or whisper on a long life course'. Dr Curson's response to this was 'how big a nudge, how often, from whom and how much should each nudge cost?'. These are important questions and addiction nurses need to know how to respond.

REFERENCES

Advisory Council on the Misuse of Drugs (1982) *Treatment and Rehabilitation*, HMSO, London.

Cochrane, R.M.C. (1989) *A Sense of Security*, Cornerstone, Maidstone Kent.

Curson, D. (1991) Attacks Exaggerated but Questions Asked. *British Medical Journal*, **86**(1), 21–3.

Donmall, M., Webster, A., Strang, J. and Tantrum, D. (1989) *The Introduction of Community Based Services for Drug Misusers*, University of Manchester Drug Research Unit, Manchester.

Dufficy, H. and Hager, K. (1993) *Standard Setting in Audit*, SCODA, London.

Gillam, S., Dubois-Arber, F., Stirzacker, L., Croft, A. and Gupta, N.D. (1992) *Public Health*, **106**(3), 209–15.

Greenwood, J. (1992) Persuading General Practitioners to Prescribe – Good Husbandry or a Recipe for Chaos? *British Journal of Addiction*, **87**(4), 567–75.

Ovretveit, J. (1992) *Health Service Quality – An Introduction to Quality Methods for Health Services*, Blackwell Science, Oxford.

Power, R., Dale, A. and Jones, S. (1991) Towards a Process Evaluation Model for Community Based Initiatives Aimed at Preventing the Spread of HIV Amongst Injecting Drug Users. *AIDS Care*, **3**, 2.

Spratley, T. (1991) The Importance of Teamwork. *Druglink*, **6**(1), 16–7.

Staff, A.J. (1993) Has Pragmatic Euphoria Undermined the Gospel of Good Health? *Association of Nurses in Substance Abuse Journal*, Issue 13.

Strang, J. and Clement, S. (1994) The Introduction of Community Drug Teams Across the UK, in *Heroin and Drug Policy – The British System* (eds J. Strang and M. Gossop), Oxford University Press, Oxford, *Tackling Drugs Together* (1995), HMSO, London.

Waller, T. (1993) *Working With General Practitioners*, Institute for the Study of Drug Dependence, London.

Wilson, A. (1992) *Evaluation of North Manchester Community Drugs Team*, North Manchester Health Authority, Manchester.

PART SIX

Professional and personal development

Professional education and training

23

G. Hussein Rassool

INTRODUCTION

The central themes that guide the professional development of addiction nurses, as specialist practitioners, are based upon their educational preparation and clinical supervision. The changes in healthcare needs and the widespread misuse of psychoactive substances in the general population demand a workforce that is skilled in nursing interventions; and capable of providing consultation and specialist care to substance misusers and their families. Due to the changes in registration and professional development (UKCC, 1994) coupled with current policy, Health of the Nation (Department of Health, 1992) and *Tackling Drugs Together* (HMSO, 1995), and educational initiatives (ENB, 1995a), addiction nurses must engage in continuing education and professional development as a statutory requirement to maintain their professional competence. The issue of clinical supervision must also be addressed in clinical practice. Chapter 24 examines the concept of clinical supervision in addiction nursing.

This chapter will briefly address key areas of policy and professional development in nursing and examines the current recommendations on education and training of both generic and specialist workers in substance misuse and addictive behaviour. An outline of the planning of training to non-specialist workers as part of the role of the practitioners is also provided.

PROFESSIONAL DEVELOPMENT

The reforms in education and professional development of nurses and the market-oriented changes in the NHS in the late 1980s have focused on the expectation that nurses and other healthcare professionals should seek the appropriate knowledge, skills and expertise to acquire professional competence. The key areas underpinning the changes include the need for professional competence and accountability and this is reflected in several documentations.

The UKCC code of professional conduct (UKCC, 1992a) for the nurse, midwife and health visitor states that 'each registered nurse, midwife and health visitor is accountable for his or her practice, and in the exercise of professional accountability shall take every reasonable opportunity to maintain and improve professional knowledge and competence'. The latest development in the continuum of reform for nursing and midwifery education is the UKCCs report on the *Standards for Education and Practice following Registration* (UKCC, 1994). The report states that 'Nurses, midwives and health visitors practise in an environment which is subject to change – in relation to the organization of services, the boundaries and delivery of healthcare and technological advances in treatment and care... The continuing demands and complexity of professional practice requires registered practitioners to not only maintain and develop their professional knowledge and competence, but to do so in the interests of patient and client care'. Thus, nurse practitioners are required to be accountable for their decisions and actions for the quality of care they provide. It is acknowledged that professional education is a requirement to the services and patients or clients for the quality and standards of educational preparation of practitioners.

The notion of professional education as a lifelong learning process is echoed in the report on *Creating Lifelong Learners* (ENB, 1994a). The report states that education for registration would enable nurses, midwives and health visitors to acquire a zest for learning. Nurses, midwives and health visitors who have developed as lifelong learners as a result of their pre-registration education have the characteristics that the ever changing health services need. Such practitioners, according to the report, are the key to enable health service purchasers and providers to achieve their strategic and operational objectives in the provision of high standards of patient and client care.

The ENB framework of higher awards (ENB, 1994) has been instrumental in changing the pattern and delivery of continuing education and has enabled the creation of a 'culture where education directly responds to the service needs while at the same time enabling individual practitioners to fulfil their ambitions'. In future, all registered nurses will have to maintain their own professional development within their own area of practice. It is through personal professional practice that all nurses will assess critically their clinical practice and identify their own professional continuing education needs (Barriball *et al.*, 1992).

The UKCCs report 'Standards for Education and Practice following Registration' (UKCC, 1994) is the latest reform in the development of continuing education for nurses and midwives. Currently, all practitioners are required to maintain effective registration by:

• completion of five study days every three years;

- completion of a 'Notification of Practice' form every three years;
- maintaining a personal professional profile;
- completion of a 'Return to Practice' programme if there has been a break from practice of five years or more.

The UKCC will require individual practitioners, including nurses working in the addiction field, to maintain a personal professional profile as a record of their professional development. They will need to show how they have fulfilled the council's requirements for five days of study and this should be updated every three years. Individual practitioners are required to record their specific learning objectives for the continuing education programmes, keep evidence that they had attended educational programmes, and record their learning outcomes and reflective practice.

The implementation of the UKCCs policy on 'Standards for Education and Practice' (UKCC, 1994) is based on 10 key characteristics (ENB, 1994) which form a framework for identification of expert practice (Table 23.1).

Table 23.1 Ten key characteristics (ENB)

- Professional accountability and responsibility
- Clinical expertise with a specific client group
- Use of research to plan, implement and evaluate
- Teamwork and leadership
- Innovative approaches to care
- Use of health promotion strategies
- Facilitating staff development
- Resource management
- Setting standards and evaluating quality of care
- Initiating, managing and evaluating clinical change

The 10 key characteristics provide a framework for practitioners to examine the range and scope of their practice. The individual practitioner can use the framework to integrate and direct continuing education programmes so that their professional statutory requirements are met. In addition, the ENB higher award is awarded to practitioners who have demonstrated their professional competence in integrating all 10 key characteristics into their practice and mastery of the learning outcomes. The ENB higher award offers professional and academic recognition for clinical practice.

POLICY DEVELOPMENT INITIATIVES

This section will review the literature relating to government strategy and advisory bodies' policy development and recommendations on substance misuse education. The prevailing political climate towards substance misuse has provided an impetus for several policies and educational initiatives in the prevention, treatment and rehabilitation of substance misusers.

The role of addiction nurses and other generic healthcare professionals is likely to augment especially in response to the targets on drugs, alcohol, HIV and sexual behaviour as outlined in the Government's Health of the Nation documents (Department of Health, 1993; 1994). The reports recommend that professional bodies in health and social work continue to design training in the early identification of alcohol misuse and appropriate referral skills and that specialist practitioners should provide training in substance misuse for professionals working in healthcare and other settings. A new strategic document on the 'war against drugs' that has underlying implications for healthcare professionals is the White Paper *Tackling Drugs Together: A Strategy for England 1995–1998*. The aim of the government's strategy is 'to take effective action by vigorous law enforcement, accessible treatment and a new emphasis on education and prevention'. This comprehensive initiative and approach to tackle the problem of substance misuse has a clear focus on education and prevention strategies and involves a co-ordinated approach both locally and nationally.

The Advisory Council on the Misuse of Drugs (ACMD) was established under the Misuse of Drugs Act, 1971. This advisory council has become the single most influential body in British drug policy and practice (Aston, 1994). Several reports: ACMD (1982;1984; 1988; 1989; 1990), Advisory Committee on Alcoholism (1978), Alcohol Concern (1994), ENB (1992), WHO/ICN (1991) and the WHO, 1993) have highlighted the need for the adequate preparation of professionals in health and social care and the criminal justice system to work with substance misusers. Chapter 16 gives an exposition of the criminal justice system and substance misuse.

The ACMD report on *Problem Drug Use: A Review of Training* (ACMD, 1990) recommended a 'three-tiered' approach to the development of a framework for professional education in substance misuse and addictive behaviour, and the expansion of training provision on 'substance problems' rather than drugs and alcohol. In relation to advanced training for specialist practitioners, the report recommended that appropriate academic institutions, in conjunction with national bodies, should devise suitable programmes for part-time courses in addiction or substance problem studies. In the alcohol field, the working group involved in the report on *A National Alcohol Training Strategy* (Alcohol Concern, 1994), recommended the urgent need for clear guidelines to be developed and introduced for education and training in substance misuse. It further added that a national forum be convened for professional bodies responsible for professional education and training to review present training requirements in alcohol misuse both in basic training for generic staff and in post basic training for specialists.

In its recommendations for nurses in relation to substance abuse, the WHO/ICN (1991) document states that nurses should be educated about substance misuse, starting at the basic training levels, and that continuing education and training should be provided for those working in this field. Furthermore, it is stated that education and training must be an integral part of service planning for all areas of treatment, and include specialist and non-specialist personnel (WHO, 1993). However, it is a pity that nationally there is a diversified educational strategy in the delivery of courses. Both educational standardization and quality are varied. The paucity of a substance misuse component in the nursing curriculum and the low priority accorded to both policy and educational development in this area have been reinforced in a recent document from the substance misuse project 'Meeting the Education and Training Needs of Nurses, Midwives and Health Visitors in the field of Substance Misuse' (ENB, 1995a).

CURRENT STATUS OF EDUCATIONAL PROGRAMMES

The ENB Report (1995a) presents the findings of the training needs analysis (TNA) of nurses, midwives and health visitors in the field of substance misuse, and outlines a strategy to implement the findings. However, the findings are, unfortunately, not encouraging. The report indicates that 'the education and training of nurses, midwives and health visitors in substance misuse is at present inadequate at pre- and post-registration levels and does not facilitate the development of knowledge, skills and attitudes necessary for caring for people with substance misuse-related problems'. There seems to be a lack of consistency in curriculum content, at both pre-and post-registration levels, which poorly reflects the current awareness of the extent and nature of the problems. Even when the content of substance misuse is included, the curriculum is restricted to the pharmacological effects of psychoactive substances. It is a pity that, even with the advent and implementation of project 2000 – pre-registration nursing courses (UKCC, 1986), the profession has made little progress in the integration of substance misuse in the health sciences curricula (Rassool, 1996).

It is encouraging to note that the ENB (1995b) at a meeting in July 1995, ratified the report and recommended that 'substance misuse be included in all pre-registration and post-registration nursing, midwifery and health visiting curricula guidelines, at a standard appropriate to each programme'. The *Guidelines for good practice in education and training of nurses, midwives and health visitors* on substance use and misuse have been published (ENB, 1996). This is a welcome mandate for the recognition of the integration of this specialty at all curricula levels. However, there appears to be some degree of confusion about whether a substance curriculum, at pre-registration level, should be an integral part of the core content or an additional module on substance misuse that is added to the already overcrowded curricula (Rassool, 1996). Rassool and Oyefeso (1993a) have suggested that in order to meet the learning needs of students, at pre-registration levels, a vertical integration model should be adopted. This approach focuses on teaching aspects of drug, alcohol and tobacco in conjunction with the content of nursing or health studies curricula.

Continuing education for addiction nurses

The relevance and importance of continuing education and training for addiction nurses have been repeatedly asserted throughout the literature. With the advent of the implementation of the UKCCs preparation for education and practice (UKCC, 1994) and the ENBs report on *Creating Lifelong Learners* (ENB, 1994), specialist nurse practitioners working in the addiction field need the specialist professional education to meet the changing nature in the use and misuse of psychoactive substances. In a recent position paper, the ENB (1995a) called for an increase in the education and training of specialist nurses in the addiction field.

Guidelines on aims and a broad indicative content of the curriculum in substance misuse education and addiction studies have been outlined. The ACMD report (1990) recommended that specialist training should equip those who are directly involved in the management of drug-related problems to embrace a whole range of knowledge and skills, including interventions, counselling, knowledge of drink/drugs interaction, research and evaluation. The practitioners should also have a solid theoretical background on the theories of substance misuse and addictive behaviour. The ENB has also provided outline curricula for their education programmes in substance misuse for generic and specialist healthcare professionals. The ENB working group, set up in response to the ACMD report (1990), reviewed the existing curricula and found that the submission documents did not address fundamental changes in the substance misuse and addictive behaviour as the result of the association of HIV/AIDS with sexual and injecting drug behaviours. The working group recommended that a substance misuse project should be established to identify the education and training needs of nurses, midwives and health visitors and should implement a strategy to promote the development of substance misuse education in the curricula. The substance misuse project was commissioned by the ENB for two years in July 1994. A report (ENB, 1995a) on the training needs analysis for nurses and other healthcare professionals at basic and post-basic levels was published in July 1995. A review of the ENB report (1995a) is found in Rassool and McKeown (1996).

At the post-registration level, the development of education and training of clinical nurse specialists in substance misuse and addictive behaviour has been restricted to a few centres. Currently, eight educational establishments approved by the ENB to conduct courses on 'drug and alcohol dependency nursing' (course 612), 'alcohol dependency nursing' (Course 620), 'recognition and management of substance abuse' (Course 962) and the 'short course on the recognition of and nursing responses to the problem drinker'. At the end of 1995, only four educational establishments (London (2), Nottingham and Leeds) were offering these courses at certificate and/or diploma levels. An MSc course in addictive behaviour based at the Centre for Addiction Studies, Department of Addictive Behaviour, St George's Hospital Medical School (University of London) is open to graduate and non-graduate addiction nurses working in the addiction field.

CONSULTATION AND TRAINING

The role of the addiction nurse as consultant, health educator and trainer has been examined elsewhere (WHO/ICN, 1991; Rassool, 1993b; ENB, 1994; 1995a). Only key areas of the role of addiction nurses as consultant and trainer to other health-care professionals will be examined in this section. In the context of this chapter, the role of the addiction nurse as consultant is referred to as 'educational and training' consultancy. This differs, though related in its educative aspects, from clinical consultation about patient or client management and care. It is through the process of consultation and education that addiction nurse specialists have a crucial role in promoting the development of professional education and training in substance misuse and addictive behaviour for healthcare professional and other occupational groups. Both the roles of the facilitator and enabler are embedded in the consultation process.

The addiction nurse specialist, as a consultant, would provide the specialized knowledge and expertise in substance misuse and addictive behaviour to interested parties. The input to pre-registration courses in nursing and health studies should be negotiated and organized through the academic institutions or through the personnel responsible for in-service or continuing education. Guidelines on clinical and teaching standards will be provided by the ENB. Consultancy should focus on three strands.

- Curriculum planning teams or an academic board of higher educational institutions responsible for the preparation of nurses, midwives and health visitors at both pre-registration and post-registration levels.
- Curriculum planning team or an academic board of higher educational institutions responsible for the education and training of professional and occupational groups in social work, education and the criminal justice system.
- Curriculum planning team or an academic board of higher educational institutions responsible for the education and training of addiction specialist.

The provision of the context of substance misuse and the technical knowledge provided by the consultant would enable the facilitation of the integration of substance misuse component within the curricula. There is an interface between consultation and training. When consultation is provided to an organization or agency on a regular basis, it is very likely to contribute to staff training and personal development.

Addiction nurses should play a key role in the training of healthcare professionals and other allied disciplines in substance misuse and addictive behaviour. They should also promote awareness sessions on substance misuse in schools, colleges and workplaces, community groups and advocate school and work policies that support those who are affected (WHO/ICN, 1991).

The education and training sessions should be targeted to the following groups: those undertaking pre-registration courses in nursing and allied disciplines; those undertaking post-registration courses in advanced nursing and healthcare sciences;

members of the primary healthcare team; staff in non-statutory and voluntary orga-nizations; staff in the prison healthcare service and criminal justice system, occu-pational nurses; and those attending specialist addiction courses. Tober (1991) describes a framework for the 'model of change' (Prochaska and DiClemente, 1984) in determining the planning of training for different occupational groups as part of a district training strategy.

At a local level, most agencies will have an input in the training of specific occupational groups and/or multiprofessionals. There are inherent practical diffi-culties involved in human resources and competing priorities that may mitigate in developing an educational and training strategy, or in undertaking a training need analysis and the delivery of a comprehensive course. Instead, an alternative strat-egy would be to have prior consultation with the collaborative parties in the plan-ning and delivery of minimal training sessions and events. In the organization of a training session in substance misuse for healthcare professional and allied disci-plines, it is important to nurture the collaboration of the service managers, clini-cians, trainers and course participants in planning the curriculum content. It is acknowledged that, although this process is complex and time-consuming, it is invaluable in the delivering of high quality training and is service-driven.

Most education and training programmes have pursued an objective of the demystification of problem drug use focusing on three main areas; knowledge, skills and attitudes. Other areas that require urgent attention include the personal health education of the professional in relation to substance use and misuse; HIV and substance misuse; health education and preventive strategies and the educa-tion and training of healthcare professionals in the rational of licit psychoac-tive substances (Ghodse and Khan, 1989; WHO, 1989,1992; Rassool et al., 1993c).

Training in substance misuse and addictive behaviour will concentrate on spe-cific knowledge and skills relevant to the particular discipline. Principles of good practice in education and training and the design and delivery of training and learning outcomes for nurses, midwives and health visitors should be adhered to in accordance with the ENBs documentations. The kind of training where most addiction nurses are likely to have an input would be short sessions included in existing courses or training events and staff development. A few others may be part of a multiprofessional team delivering professionally accredited courses in substance misuse. The role of substance misuse specialists as multiprofessional trainers should be continued and their input into ENB recognized programmes rec-ommended in curricula (ENB, 1995a, 1996).

CONCLUSION

In this chapter the emphasis has been on the importance of professional education and development in aspects of addiction nursing. Professional development will always be most effective when it is part of a strategic plan to create an organizational learning culture. It is argued that the dual development and integration of substance misuse curriculum at pre-registration and post-registration levels should be part of a parallel process of change (Rassool, 1996). If education and training in addiction for all healthcare professionals are to become a reality, policy makers, professional associations, educationalists and clinicians need to capitalize on the current political climate to focus on an effective strategy for enhancing substance misuse education on the professional agenda.

REFERENCES

Advisory Committee on Alcoholism (1978) *The Pattern and Range of Services for Problem Drinkers*, HMSO, London.

Advisory Council for the Misuse of Drugs (1982) *Treatment and Rehabilitation*, HMSO, London.

Advisory Council for the Misuse of Drugs (1984) *Prevention*, HMSO, London.

Advisory Council for the Misuse of Drugs (1988) *Aids and Drug Misuse, Part 1*, HMSO, London.

Advisory Council for the Misuse of Drugs (1989) *Aids and Drug Misuse, Part 2*, HMSO, London.

Advisory Council on the Misuse of Drugs (1990) *Problem Drug Use: A Review of Training*, HMSO, London.

Alcohol Concern (1994) *A National Alcohol Training Strategy*, Alcohol Concern, London.

Aston, M. (1994) The power of persuasion. *Druglink*, **9**, 5.

Barriball, K.L., While, A. and Norman, I.J. (1992) Continuing professional education for qualified nurse: a review of the literature. *Journal of Advanced Nursing*, **17**(9), 1129–40.

Department of Health (1992) *The Health of the Nation: A Strategy for Health in England*, HMSO, London.

Department of Health (1993) *A Vision for the Future. The Nursing, Midwifery and Health Visiting Contribution to Health and Healthcare*, HMSO, London.

Department of Health (1994) *Working in Partnership: A Collaborative Approach to Care: A Report of the Mental Health Review Team*, HMSO, London.

English National Board for Nursing, Midwifery and Health Visiting (1992) *Final Report of Working Group on The Education and Training Needs of Nurses Working in the Field of Substance Misuse*, ENB, London.

English National Board for Nursing, Midwifery and Health Visiting (1994) *Creating Lifelong Learners – Partnerships for Care*, ENB, London.

English National Board for Nursing, Midwifery and Health Visiting (1995a) *Training Needs Analysis*, ENB, London.

English National Board for Nursing, Midwifery and Health Visiting (1995b) *Press Release, July*, ENB, London.

English National Board for Nursing, Midwifery and Health Visiting (1996) *Substance use and misuse: Guidelines for good practice in education and training of nurses, midwives and health visitors*, ENB, London.

Ghodse, A.H. and Khan, I. (1988) *Psychoactive Drugs: Improving Prescribing Practices*, World Health Organization, Geneva.

Prochaska, J. and DiClemente, C. (1984) *The Transtheoretical Approach: Crossing*

Traditional Boundaries of Therapy, Dow Jones, Irwin, Homewood, IL.

Rassool, G.H. and Oyefeso, A. (1993a) The need for substance misuse education in health studies curriculum: a case for nursing education. *Nurse Education Today*, **13**(2), 107–10.

Rassool, G.H. (1993b) Substance Misuse: Responding to the Challenge. *Journal of Advanced Nursing*, **18**(9), 1401–7.

Rassool, G.H. and Winnington, J. (1993c) Using Psychoactive Drugs. *Nursing Times*, **89**(47), 38–40.

Rassool, G.H. and McKeown, O. (1996) A Review of the Report on the Education and Training of Health Care in Substance Misuse: Complacency or Commitment? *Journal of Substance Misuse*, **1**(2), 114–15.

Rassool, G.H. (1996) Editorial. Addiction Nursing and Substance Misuse: A Slow Response to Partial Accommodation. *Journal of Advanced Nursing*, **24**(2), 425–27.

Tackling Drugs Together: A Strategy for England 1995–1998 (1995) HMSO, London.

Tober, G. (1991) *Formulating Regional Training Strategies*. Paper presented at Training Excellence Conference, University of Canterbury, Kent.

United Kingdom Central Council for Nursing, Midwifery and Health Visiting (1986) *Project 2000: A New Preparation for Practice*, UKCC, London.

United Kingdom Central Council for Nursing, Midwifery and Health Visiting (1992a) *Code of Conduct for the Nurse, Midwife and Health Visitor*, UKCC, London.

United Kingdom Central Council for Nursing, Midwifery and Health Visiting (1992b) *The Scope of Professional Practice*, UKCC, London.

United Kingdom Central Council for Nursing, Midwifery and Health Visiting (1994) *The future of Professional Practice: The Council's Standards for Education and Practice Following Registration*, UKCC, London.

World Health Organization (1989) *Report on the WHO meeting of Nursing and Midwifery Education on the Rationale Use of Psychoactive Drugs (MNH/PAD)*, WHO, Geneva.

World Health Organization (1992) *Progress Report by the Director-General*, WHO A45/7, Geneva.

World Health Organization/International Council of nurses (1991) *Nurses responding to Substance Abuse*, WHO/ICN, Geneva.

World Health Organization (1993) *Expert Committee on Drug Dependence*, 28th Report, WHO, Geneva.

Clinical supervision
24

G. Hussein Rassool

INTRODUCTION

There is a growing awareness of the need for clinical supervision as an essential element in the development of professional competence in nursing practice. Addiction nurses, like any other nurse specialists, are envisaged to be autonomous practitioners with professional competence in the delivery of care and accountable to the clients and the profession. Faugier (1994) suggests that extended clinical practice, increased autonomous practice and a greater degree of responsibility for decision-making have combined to increase awareness of the need for clinical supervision.

Several reports have highlighted the importance of clinical supervision and recommended that nurses, midwives and health visitors should embrace the concept of clinical supervision and incorporate it as an integral part of their practice: Department of Health (1993, 1994), UKCC (1995) and the ENB (1995). Faugier (1994) argues that, despite increasing recognition of the importance of clinical supervision, few mental health nurses have access to skilled, sensitive and formal supervision.

Those who work in a developmental nursing specialty such as addiction nursing have derived a need for clinical supervision because of the nature of their work within a multidisciplinary framework and the multiple roles they operate. In some areas of mental health nursing, including addiction nursing, the model of clinical supervision used has been based upon a multidiscplinary supervision framework as described by Thomas and Reid (1995).

The reality of clinical supervision is that it is seldom clear-cut in the context of addiction nursing and substance misuse. Staff (Chapter 22) states that 'the opportunity for independent autonomous working practices in a specialism where the patient or client group is frequently operating in an illegal underworld or subculture is a danger... and becoming over involved, overstresses or stretches the boundaries of professional conduct'. Clinical supervision as a priority for nurses in the substance misuse field can no longer be ignored.

This chapter examines the concept, purposes and forms of clinical supervision. An outline of the models of clinical supervision is presented and criteria for choosing a supervisor briefly described. Finally, the chapter includes discussion of a pilot study on the perceptions of addiction nurses towards clinical supervision.

WHAT IS CLINICAL SUPERVISION?

The definitions of supervision are many, and are sometimes based on the nature of the professional discipline. These definitions are often conflicting and contradictory and this is augmented by the negative connotations attached to the concept. In its simplest form clinical supervision refers to a process of practising, experiencing and reflecting upon clinical practice. Clinical supervision can be seen as a formal process whereby a worker and an experienced practitioner meet to examine and reflect on the management of clients and the refinement of therapeutic skills.

In the context of clinical supervision in nursing, Butterworth and Faugier (1992) describe supervision as 'an exchange between practising professionals to enable the development of professional skills'. This seems to suggest that there must be a formal and a logical approach to reviewing one's professional work with a more experienced colleague. Another definition is one by Longanbill *et al.* (1982) which states that supervision is 'an intensive, interpersonally focused, one-to-one relationship in which one person is designated to facilitate the development of therapeutic competence in the other person'. The definition allows for, but does not adequately stress the importance of personal support. It omits the wider functions of educative, supportive and managerial relationship described by Kadushin (1976).

Purpose of supervision

An important and central focus of clinical supervision is to enhance the quality of services to clients or patients, and it is generally acknowledged that introducing clinical supervision into clinical practice would derive benefits for both practitioners and the client. Nurse practitioners, with the help of clinical supervision, would be able to develop professional competencies in specific areas of their work and with adequate supervision and support, stress and burnout are thus reduced. It is argued that practitioners who are well supported, up-to-date and professionally aware as a result of having access to effective clinical supervision will benefit the organization (UKCC, 1995). Moreover, it is stated that supervision has the potential to reduce litigation and complaints' levels in the NHS and to operate as an effective risk management tool (Tingle, 1995). There is also evidence to suggest that good supervision correlates with job satisfaction (Cherniss and Egnatios, 1978).

The task of supervision, according to Hawkins and Shohet (1989), is to develop the skills, understanding and ability of the supervisee, as well as other functions, depending on the settings. Kadushin (1976) describes three main roles of supervision:

- educative;
- supportive;
- managerial.

In the nursing profession it is common to have a combination of these three roles in dealing with a supervisee. This may be achieved through the system of personal tutorial (educative and support) and clinical supervision (educative, managerial and support). There is also the assertion that a good deal of supervision takes place in the areas where managerial (quality control function), supportive and educative considerations all intermingle (Hawkins and Shohet, 1989). In summary, the purpose of clinical supervision includes the maintenance of clinical standards, development of professional competence, reducing stress and burnout and provides support and good job satisfaction.

Forms of supervision

There are many forms of clinical supervision: self supervision, one-to-one, co-supervision, group supervision and peer supervision. The one-to-one supervision and group supervision are common in mental health nursing and addiction nursing.

Self supervision

This is a form of 'self-reflecting in action' that is important in personal and professional development, and it can occur in a variety of different contexts. This form of self supervision is valid to the individual; and the ability to explore our own thoughts, feelings and actions with self evaluation is seen as therapeutic. Self supervision should always be accompanied by one or other forms of supervisory practices. What is essential for all forms of self supervision is giving oneself enough time and also being willing to confront one's own ways of working with a healthy 'internal supervisor'(Kagan, 1980; Hawkins and Shohet, 1989).

One-to-one

This is the most common form of supervision that is given and received on an informal basis by practitioners in the helping profession. It is acknowledged that one-to-one clinical supervision will become a model in most branches of nursing but on a formal and regular basis. For example, a student receives clinical and academic supervision by one or more supervisors. A clinical nurse specialist provides clinical supervision to a drug and alcohol worker.

Co-supervision

As in co-counselling, co-supervision involves two practitioners. Both practition-ers alternate the role of supervisor and supervisee in providing clinical supervision for each other. This form of supervision usually occurs on an informal basis among practitioners working in the community.

Group supervision

Group supervision is common in mental health nursing and involves a supervisor or consultant external to the agency or with a different orientation being responsi-ble for the facilitation of the group. The group facilitator negotiates the allotted time with the supervisee for the presentation of case works. The consultation group can arrive at formulations and strategies that provide the group members with new understanding and action plans.

Geller (1994) asserts that group supervision augments traditional supervision and is an effective tool for teaching students about group work, thus students are sensitized to the group process as a medium for growth and change. The advan-tages of group supervision over one-to-one supervision include: cost-effectiveness in terms of time and money; supportive environment; testing out or checking emo-tional and intuitive responses with other members of the group; receiving feedback and input from group members and the facilitator; provision of a wider range of life experiences; and use of group and action techniques. However, group super-vision is less likely to mirror the dynamics of the individual session, and the dynamics of the group could become a preoccupation to members with less time for individual members to have supervision (Hawkins and Shohet, 1989).

Peer supervision

Peer supervision is common in substance misuse agencies and is conducted on an informal basis in which the multidisciplinary team shares the responsibility for providing clinical supervision within a group context. The potential problems of using only peer supervision are that current norms of practice may be perpetuated, and the exploration of innovative or alternative practices is less likely to occur (Devine and Baxter, 1995). It is argued that peer supervision is not recommended for the novice, the newly qualified practitioner or those who lack adequate skills and professional competence. In a study by Benshoff (1993) on peer supervision in counsellor training, it was found that 70 subjects out of a total sample of 81 stu-dents reported that peer supervision had been very helpful in developing their skills and the understanding of counselling concepts. However, it was also found that subjects who received peer supervision did not rate themselves higher on counselling effectiveness than those who received traditional supervision.

Models of clinical supervision – a review

The model of supervision and supervisory practices used by supervisors is largely dependent on their orientation to a particular school of counselling and psychotherapy. Some supervisors would use an integrated or eclectic model of clinical supervision based on the humanistic, psychoanalytical, transpersonal and behavioural school of psychology. Others would base their supervisory practices upon the framework and philosophical underpinnings of a particular school of psychology.

A number of models of supervision can be identified in the literature: growth and support model (Faugier, 1992); interactive model (Proctor, 1991); triadic model (Milne, 1986); multicultural model (Ramirez, 1991) and integrative model (Hawkins and Shohet, 1989). Some of the nursing based literature is descriptive of clinical supervision in the psychotherapy mode. Dombeck and Brody (1995) describe the principles and processes of a model of clinical supervision for psychotherapy by drawing heavily on Peplau's (1952) theory of interpersonal relations and Bowen's (1978) family systems theory.

Rich (1993) describes an integrated model of supervision that identifies its basic requirements. In its organizational context, in which it is embedded, clinical supervision fulfils four functions:

- facilitating a supportive learning and work environment;
- fostering staff development;
- providing a means for the professional socialization of staff;
- ensuring the delivery of effective client services.

The UKCCs statement on clinical supervision also argues that there is no single model that can be used in every clinical setting and that local practitioners will need to develop an approach that suits its particular needs.

Aspects of clinical supervision in substance misuse

This section is a brief review of the literature pertaining to clinical supervision in the substance misuse. Powell and Brodsky (1993) argue that the substance abuse field requires a model of supervision that synthesizes all the (developmental, psychodynamic, skills and family therapy) traditions into a coherent whole that reflects the principles and practices specific to alcohol and drug abuse counselling. They have designed a comprehensive, 'blended' model, and offer guidelines for its use with substance abuse workers and counsellors.

The reader may find the following selected literature on aspects of supervision useful. The relevant papers are: supervision: *profile of a good clinical supervisor* (Powell, 1991); *preparing to take on clinical supervision* (Butterworth, 1994); *the implementation of clinical supervision using a case study* (Devine and Baxter, 1995); *a descriptive model of staff supervision in a community mental health home* (Oliver, 1995); *clinical supervision of psychiatric nursing students* (Adams, 1991);

clinical supervision in psychiatric nursing (Bodley, 1992); *Clinical supervision as a self-actualizing process* (Farkas-Cameron, 1995); *role of clinical supervision in mental health practice* (Morris, 1995); *multidisciplinary clinical supervision in mental health* (Thomas and Reid, 1995); and *supervision of substance misuse counsellors and therapists* (Todd and Heath, 1992).

Choosing a supervisor

It is acknowledged that a novice practitioner should always be mentored by an advanced practitioner, that is, the less experienced should be supervized by an experienced and competent practitioner. Supervisors in nursing and other health-care profession should have a first level registration as well as formal educational preparation in clinical supervision. The process of supervision depends very much on the supervisor and supervisee's levels of motivation, development and past experiences of supervision.

Watkins (1995) reviewed four models of supervisor development and found that all supervisors begin in a state of uncertainty, insecurity, anxiety and inexperience. They wrestle with various issues; progress by means of time, experience, and struggle; and ultimately forge a supervisory identity and become competent. According to Devine and Baxter (1995) the supervisor should adhere to the following criteria:

- receive supervision;
- have some form of preparation;
- be RN trained or have identifiable skills/qualifications;
- demonstrate facilitation skills;
- be a reflective and proactive practitioner;
- be chosen by supervisee;
- be willing to give supervision;
- understand the privilege of the position;
- be worthy of respect, respect confidentiality;
- utilize research findings.

However, it is the supervisor's skills and expertise in conveying the relevance of his/her experience to the supervisee that are of prime importance (Kohner, 1994). There are, however, organizational factors and inherent ambiguities in this managerial relationship and supervisory situation where conflicts may inhibit the learning process. Contemporary clinical supervision in nursing and allied professions has focused heavily on management accountability and quality control and less on other aspects in teaching and consultation. The UKCC (1994) has stated 'that clinical supervision should not be an exercise of managerial responsibility and managerial supervision, nor a system of formal individual performance review procedures or hierarchical'. The choice of having a line manager as supervisor can lead to difficulties, since a conflict of interests may arise between the needs of the substance misuse agencies and the needs of the supervisee. The UKCCs position statement on clinical supervision states that practitioners should have a say in who acts as their clinical supervisor, and although the supervisor will normally be a registered nurse, it is possible to have a clinician from another profession in exceptional cases. This is applicable for addiction nurses as in many community-oriented substance misuse teams there may be only one nurse as a full member of the team.

Perception of addiction nurses

There is an assumption that nurses are generally inclined to embrace and to receive clinical supervision. Hawkins and Shohet (1989) identified interpersonal, organizational and professional factors that may make individuals reluctant to give and receive supervision. These barriers may be applicable to addiction nurses and include:

- previous experience of supervision;
- personal inhibitions;
- difficulties in the supervisory relationship;
- organizational blocks;
- practical block;
- culture of the organization;
- the profession's being antithetical to supervision.

Nurses' beliefs and attitudes are highly significant towards the positive acceptance of clinical supervision as an integral part of professional practice. There is a paucity of literature on the attitudes of nurses towards clinical supervision, and few studies on the nature of clinical supervision in mental health nursing. Persut et al., (1990) administered the 'nursing clinical supervision questionnaire' to 61 clinical nurse specialists and found that supervision seemed to be highly valued, although many did not feel well prepared to assume the role of the clinical supervisor. There were disagreements on such items as structuring the supervisory session.

A pilot study (Rassool 1995) was undertaken to explore and examine the perception of addiction nurses towards clinical supervision. An opportunistic sample of 20 addiction nurses completed a self-reported questionnaire – 'clinical supervision perception questionnaire' (CSPQ). A focus group was also used to elicit further content and themes regarding clinical supervision. Only key preliminary findings of the study, which is still in progress at the time of writing, will be presented in the next section. The sample consists of 13 females (65%) and 7 males (35%).

The result shows that 85% of the subjects believe that supervision is good for professional practice and 65% think that supervision should be compulsory for all practitioners. When asked about the appropriateness and the adequacy of clinical supervision, 50% agree with the statement and 30% think that the supervisions they received were not adequate at all. 85% agreed that supervision made them feel more confident in their abilities and skills and made them aware of their strengths and limitations. The types of supervision that were employed were: one-to-one supervision (65%) and case supervision (60%). Only 20% of the subjects reported having group supervision.

There is a commonly held view that clinical supervision is not very different to other support systems and this finding supports existing literature (Fox, 1995). It seemed that one-to-one clinical supervision is more popular with practitioners, as this form of supervision offers the potential to separate appraisal and clinical work. In summary, this pilot study does indicate that addiction nursing practitioners are receiving clinical supervision on a regular basis and that they believe supervision has improved their professional competence.

CONCLUSION

If clinical supervision is to remain an integral part of the lifelong learning process, there is a need to develop standardized training and clinical standards in practice. There are few studies that examine directly the relationships of the supervisee performance and its relations to patient outcomes. There is a need for a shared understanding of the tasks and purposes of clinical supervision in nursing, especially for those undertaking undergraduate professional courses. Although some form of supervision is grounded in mental health nursing, it remains underdeveloped in the addiction field. Existing models of supervision, either integrated or developmental models of clinical supervision could be adapted to fulfil the gap in supervision framework and delivery. The agenda and action of clinical supervision in addiction nursing remain with clinicians, educators and managers to provide an organizational culture whereby clinical supervision could flourish. It is hoped that clinical supervision as a developmental activity, in the substance misuse field, would generate more research. The focus should be based not only on the effectiveness of educational programmes but also on whether improvement of professional competence, as a result of supervision, has a direct benefit for the client in the delivery of quality care.

REFERENCES

Adams, T. (1991) Clinical supervision: psychiatric students. *Nursing Standard*, 5(26), 29–31.

Benshoff, J. (1993) Peer supervision in counsellor training. *Clinical Supervisor*, 11(2), 89–102.

Bodley, D.E. (1992) Clinical Supervision in psychiatric nursing: using the process record. *Nurse Education Today*, 12(2), 148–55.

Bowen, M. (1978) *Family Therapy in Clinical Practice*, Aronson, New York.

Butterworth, T. (1994) Preparing to take on clinical supervision. *Nursing Standard*, 8(52), 32–4.

Butterworth, T. and Faugier J. (eds) (1992) *Clinical Supervision and Mentorship in Nursing*, Chapman & Hall, London.

Cherniss, C. and Egnatios, E. (1978) Clinical Supervision in Community Mental Health. *Social Work*, **23**(2), 219–23.

Department of Health (1993) *A Vision for the Future. The Nursing, Midwifery and Health Visiting Contribution to Health and Healthcare*, HMSO, London.

Department of Health (1994) *Working in Partnership: A Review of Mental Health Nursing*, HMSO, London.

Devine, A. and Baxter, D. (1995) Introducing Clinical Supervision: A Guide. *Nursing Standard*, **9**(40), 32–4.

Dombeck, M.T. and Brody, S.L. (1995) Clinical Supervision: A Three-Way Mirror. *Archives of Psychiatric Nursing*, **9**(1), 3–10.

English National Board for Nurses, Midwives and Health Visitors (1989) *Preparation of Teachers, Practitioner/Teachers, Mentors and Supervisors in the context of Project 2000*, ENB, London.

English National Board for Nurses, Midwives and Health Visitors (1995) *The Board's Response to Working in Partnership: a Collaborative Approach To Care*, ENB, London.

Farkas-Cameron, M.M. (1995) Clinical Supervision in Psychiatric Nursing: a self-actualizing process. *Journal of Psychosocial Nursing and Mental Health Services*, **33**(2), 31–9.

Faugier, J. (1992) The supervisory relationship, in *Clinical Supervision and Mentorship in Nursing* (eds C.A. Butterworth and J. Faugier), Chapman & Hall, London.

Faugier, J. (1994) Thin on the ground ... clinical supervision in mental health nursing. *Nursing Times*, **90**(20), 64–5.

Fox, P. (1995) Nursing Developments: Trust nurses' views. *Nursing Standard*, **9**(18), 31–4.

Geller, C. (1994) Group supervision as a vehicle for teaching group work to students: Field instruction in a senior center. Special Issue: Field instruction in social work settings. *Clinical Supervisor,* **12**(1), 199–214.

Hawkins, P. and Shohet, R. (1989) *Supervising in the Helping Professions*, Open University Press, Milton Keynes.

Hess, A.K. (ed.) (1980) *Psychotherapy Supervision: Theory, Research and Practice*, Wiley, New York.

Kadushin, A. (1976) *Supervision in Social Work*, Columbia University Press, New York.

Kagan, N. (1980) Influencing human interaction – eighteen years with IPR, in *Psychotherapy Supervision: Theory, Research and Practice* (ed. A.K. Hess), Wiley, New York.

Kohner, N. (1994) *Clinical Supervision in Practice*, King's Fund Centre, London.

Loganbill, C., Hardy, H. And Delworth, U. (1982) Supervision: a conceptual model. *Counselling Psychologist,* **10**, 3–42.

Milne, D. (1986) *Training Behaviour Therapists: Methods, Evaluation and Implementation with Parents, Nurses and Teachers*, Brookline, Cambridge.

Morris, M. (1995) The role of clinical supervision in mental health practice. *British Journal of Nursing*, **4**(15), 886–88.

Oliver, J. (1995) Central support ... a system of clinical supervision. *Nursing Times*, **9**(26), 32–3.

Peplau, H. (1952) *Interpersonal Relations in Nursing*, Putnam, New York.

Pesut, D.J. and Williams, C.A. (1990) The nature of clinical supervision in psychiatric nursing: A survey of clinical specialists. *Archives of Psychiatric Nursing*, **4**(3), 188–94.

Powell, D.J. and Brodsky, A. (1993) *Clinical supervision in alcohol and drug abuse counselling: Principles, models and methods*. Lexington Books/ Macmillan Inc., New York.

Powell, D.J. (1991) Supervision: Profile of a clinical supervisor. *Alcoholism Treatment Quarterly*, **8**(1), 69–86.

Proctor, B. (1991) On Being a Trainer, in *Training and Supervision for Counselling in Action* (eds W. Dryden and B. Thorne), Sage, London.

Ramirez III, M. (1991) *Psychotherapy and Counselling with minorities: A Cognitive Approach to Individual and Cultural Differences*, Pergamon press, London.

Rassool, G.H. (1995) Perception of Addiction Nurses towards Clinical Supervision. Centre for Addiction Studies, Department of Addictive Behaviour, St George's Hospital Medical School. (Unpublished paper).

Rich, P. (1993) The form function and content of clinical supervision: An integrated model. *Clinical Supervisor*, **11**(1), 137–78.

Stoltenberg, C.D. and Delworth, U. (1987) *Supervising Counsellors and Therapists*, Josey Bass, San Francisco.

Thomas, B. and Reid, J. (1995) Multidisciplinary clinical supervision. *British Journal of Nursing*, **4**(15), 803–5.

Tingle, J. (1995) Clinical Supervision is an effective risk management tool. *British Journal of Nursing*, **4**(14), 794–5.

Todd, T.C. and Heath A.W. (1992) Supervision of substance abuse counsellors, in *Handbook for assessing and treating addictive disorders* (eds C.E. Stout, J.L. Levitt and H.R. Douglas), Greenwood Press, New York.

United Kingdom Central Council for Nursing, Midwifery and Health Visiting (1994) *The future of Professional Practice: The Council's Standards for Education and Practice Following Registration*, UKCC, London.

United Kingdom Central Council for Nursing, Midwifery and Health Visiting (1995) *Clinical Supervision for Nursing and Health Visiting*, Registrar's letter, 4/95, 24 January. UKCC, London.

Watkins, C.E. (1995) Psychotherapy supervisor development: On Musings, models and metaphor. *Journal of Psychotherapy Practice and Research*, **4**(2), 150–8.

Projects and research: an agenda for action

25

Stephen Byrne and Bridget Kilpatrick

INTRODUCTION

Research is described as 'seeking through methodical processes to add to one's own body of knowledge and, hopefully, to that of others, by the discovery of non-trivial facts and insights' (Howard and Sharp, 1989). The opportunity to undertake projects or research has not been a major influence upon why people choose to enter the nursing profession. Nursing skills may be viewed by many, both within and outside the profession, as usefully directed towards the nursing care of patients. Despite recent changes to the structure, functioning and current practices within the health service which have given nurses additional tasks and responsibilities, such as the expanded role, research remains a topic viewed as distant, unfamiliar and underused. Moreover, professional responsibility, the growth of specialist clinical practice and changes within nurse education and the promotion of academic standards during initial and subsequent training have contributed to research becoming an integral part of current work practice or continued training. While the *Report of the Mental Health Nursing Review Team* (Department of Health, 1994) does not require all mental health nurses to be participating in, or undertaking research, the review of mental health nursing recently undertaken does expect nurses to be familiar with the processes of research.

In the early 1980s it was usual for one community psychiatric nurse to have been working as the sole designated nurse in a district providing care to substance misusers. At that time support, supervision and training were the important issues to establish, and undertaking addiction research was generally not considered.

There is now wide variety in the provision of care for the substance misuser. Nurses are found in assessment, treatment, counselling and rehabilitation settings that offer opportunities to those interested and willing to undertake addiction research projects in the course of patient care. Nurses have become a well-represented profession working within institutional and community substance misuse services (MacGregor *et al.*, 1991). Drug misusers are frequently brought into contact with the criminal justice system; either directly as a result of their misuse of controlled drugs or because their misuse of drugs caused or contributed to their offence. Nurses working within the prison system encounter the problems of substance misuse and those working in community drug services often care for drug misusers receiving probation or other community based sentences. The non-statutory sector offers addiction nurses, working in or seconded to such agencies, further opportunities to extend nursing skills. Nurses are represented as practitioners across the range of interventions and treatments, and thus are in an excellent position to undertake a project, whether as part of a local study, diploma or degree which combines the utilization of formal research skills and clinical contact with the substance misuser.

This chapter relates to the experiences of two addiction research nurses, drawing upon some of these prevailing changes, the debates within nursing and research aspects relating to substance misuse. The development of a model for research is offered as an introduction to undertaking a project. Further directions in research and its role within nursing in the future are discussed in the final section.

PERSPECTIVES OF NURSING RESEARCH

There is a certain lack of clarity about the title 'research nurse'; what is involved and what is implied by this term. Are research nurses researchers or nurses? It is arguable that in some cases the term nurse is an inappropriate one because of the small amount, or absence, of clinical nursing content in their research role. It is perhaps similar to the situation faced by nurse lecturers – are they primarily educators or nurse teachers? In both examples there are those who would wish to keep their identity as nurses.

What then are the particular qualities required of the research nurse? It could be their knowledge, familiarity or expertise in a particular field of nursing, their research training and experience or a combination of both practices. This raises the question of whether experience of a particular methodological tradition of research is necessary or whether research skills can be acquired and applied in many clinical settings. One definite contribution that the nurse, as a researcher, can bring into the field of research is that of understanding and relating to, in a professional manner, patients who are research subjects. The 'subject' may also express concerns or ask questions that are best dealt with by someone with experience or understanding of the matter in hand. A nurse researcher may be well placed to fill this role, providing a bridge between nursing care and research. Research nurses with experience of particular clinical areas can also provide valuable teaching input into training courses.

In an ideal world the implementation of nursing research would play an everyday part in nursing practice, in terms of both carrying out research and in integrating research findings into daily practice. Whether or not this is the case is open to discussion. We have all experienced wards of which 'the land where time stood still' would be an apt description, places where research is at best ignored and at worst reviled. Fortunately they seem to be a disappearing phenomenon as nurses are under increasing pressure to keep up to date in their knowledge and practice.

Interest in research should be encouraged at the earliest stages of a nursing career, that is to say while a student. Basic training in research methodology will become essential for all nurses if the future of nursing is to lie in research-based practice. Even if not directly involved in research, a nurse will need to be able to evaluate the research of others. The requirements of post-registration education and practice (UKCC, 1994) accentuate this need, placing as it does on all nurses the responsibility to continually update their skills and knowledge.

Developments in nursing roles

The role of the nurse is currently undergoing change. Many of the traditional 'hands on' roles are being delegated to less skilled or trained personnel and some of the tasks previously within a medical remit are becoming a nursing responsibility. The important role of the addiction nurse as educator or manager has already been accepted, a change increasingly reflected in training. Is it not feasible therefore for the nurse as researcher to become equally integrated into the model of nursing practice? Pre- and post-registration students are exhorted to undertake small scale projects: surveys, literature reviews and patient interviews as part of their training, using skills central to research. With appropriate supervision and support there is no reason why these skills cannot continue to be incorporated and utilized in our everyday work after training is completed. The key word is supervision. To be carried out efficiently and with purpose, all research needs to be well supervised by those in a position to do so. It also requires the encouragement and support of managers who may need to be persuaded about the benefits of a particular piece of research. Primarily, this task will be up to the nurse who wishes to carry out the research.

Developing and presenting a research proposal is often a difficult aspect and necessitates sound organization prior to presentation. Colleagues may need an explanation in order to persuade them to contribute in the process of, for example, the collection of data. They will also need reassurance that this need not prevent them from continuing to carry out their own duties effectively. Recognition of such input should always be acknowledged, as their assistance is invaluable and may be valuable again in the future. It may also encourage others to undertake research.

Obtaining the goodwill and permission from nursing management to undertake research could be a different proposition. Issues such as cost effectiveness, time management and human resources, and demonstrating their relevance to service needs and effects upon the delivery of patient care will require careful thought and should be addressed prior to the presentation of a research proposal.

Research nurses, who are working full-time, are not always able to initiate their own research projects, at least in the early stages of their career. This is simply because such nurses are usually employed to carry out and participate in other planned studies, involving data collection, basic analysis and writing of reports. However this should be an opportunity to consolidate existing skills, acquire further expertise and become familiar with other aspects of the research process. Nurses working primarily as researchers can have advantages over full-time clinical nurses undertaking research as time management problems will change and commitment to clinical care is likely to be less. This raises the problem of appropriate roles for the research nurse, for the research undertaken is unlikely to include a nursing perspective. It is true, data may be obtained which can be applicable to nursing practice and a good research nurse may be able to sift and collate such data and present it in a such a way as to make it relevant to nursing perspectives and practice.

Features of substance misuse research

Research in the field of addictive behaviour does have particular difficulties. These are related to the secretive and often illegal activities involved in drug misuse. Subjects may be reluctant to talk to someone they do not know, although this can be less of a problem for the nurse as researcher who may already know their subject. Common concerns of the subject will include what use the data will be put to and fear of exposure to statutory organizations. Clear explanation of the confidentiality guidelines and scrupulous adherence to them is paramount to recruit and retain subjects. It will be necessary to explain precisely in the study proposal how this will be achieved, e.g. use of code numbers to preserve identity, where files will be kept, who will have access to them and for what purposes the information will be used. These details should be cleared with the subject at the beginning of the study. The boundaries of confidentiality can, in some circumstances, pose a problem for a researcher, in terms of what can or cannot be kept secret and from whom. For example, information given in confidence as part of research could have direct implications for treatment. While limits of confidentiality may in the final analysis rest with the researcher, prior discussion about them with colleagues, supervisors and the subjects may help to avoid difficult situations and incomplete research.

During the course of investigations it may be necessary to collect details of a sensitive or highly personal nature such as those related to sexual practices, prostitution, and abuse within personal relationships. Such investigations will require a tactful and sensitive approach by an appropriate researcher who will need to reinforce explanations as to why the data is required. It cannot be assumed that subjects will give intimate details of their lives simply because a nurse requests this data however vital the research is regarded by the nurse. Consideration must be given to what the patient-subject wants from the system, and the nurse should be prepared to explain exactly how the research is relevant to the patient. Smith (1992) provides an example of research by a nurse as well as valuable discussion of some of the problems that the researcher may encounter.

Drug-taking behaviour that can be both secretive and dangerous can impose and place limits upon research. A researcher involved in a longitudinal study may find that keeping trace of subjects is problematic. Patients leaving treatment may not wish to be contacted – a patient being treated without the knowledge of the family or friends can also fall into this category. Further tracing difficulties can result from subjects moving home, being of no fixed address when interviewed, going into custody and dying. Tracing can be time-consuming and frustrating but adequate forward planning may prevent complications that could undermine the research by not having enough recruits or completed interviews.

Another difficulty affecting addiction research is the problem posed by substance misusers who do not come into contact with treatment services. The differences between those who do and do not engage in treatment have been highlighted (Ghodse, 1977), and of course it is extremely difficult to estimate these numbers. Tober (1994) suggests examining several sources in order to gain a more accurate picture of the level of drug taking activity in a district. This could include the number of drug-related incidents dealt with by accident and emergency departments (sometimes the only contact with services) or looking at the uptake of local needle and syringe exchange facilities. A word of caution needs to be expressed here about using such measures of drug use activity. All data is open to various interpretations and the skill is in making an accurate one. For example, the number of arrests for drug offences may more accurately reflect levels of police activity, or increased levels of uptake of needle and syringe exchange may result from a successful health education or harm-minimization campaign. Careful scrutiny of data and its sources at an early stage may prevent embarrassment or disaster at a later one. Never be afraid to seek a second opinion at any stage.

Addiction nurses seeking to undertake full-time research should understand that this will make a significant difference to their nursing career and should consider this carefully. This is particularly important with the current trend towards fixed term contracts. The nurse who wishes to move into research may be well advised to consider carefully what it is they wish to gain in terms of their longer-term career prospects. The prospect of whether or not to return to clinical nursing will also need careful consideration. Research experience is valuable for someone considering a move into an academic field. In common with other work experiences, the value of research experience in nursing will need to be evaluated when the time comes to seek further employment.

Model for a research project

Initial undertaking of a project will involve exposure to unfamiliar terminology, confusion over the processes and probably greater uncertainty over the types of fieldwork or methodology and analysis. These factors are encountered by all new researchers and are not insurmountable. Research into the different types of addictions does not necessarily require a separate textbook as many of the processes involved are:

- the identification of a research problem;
- review of the relevant literature;
- development of a theoretical approach;
- formulation of an initial plan of study;
- data collection and analysis;
- writing up of the research report.

However, there are particular difficulties which may be encountered in addiction research and have been referred to earlier, such as dealing with hidden or stigmatized groups, confidentiality, sensitive topics, illegal activities, uncertainty over the extent of the activity and several of these factors will influence the accuracy of some official statistics. A useful exercise to ascertain how some of these problems are overcome is to review relevant published research articles and examine other research proposals that address the highlighted problem.

Choosing a reasoned question or topic for research will involve time, background reading, thinking and re-thinking and discussion in order to arrive at a research problem. In the early phase of thinking about a topic it is possible to feel devoid of any ideas but it is important to persevere. Motives, ideas and theories are prevailing influences upon us. Interests, values, ideologies and prejudices exist in the human world. Contemporary western scientific application has derived from a belief that we find facts out by empirical thought, which contains three main characteristics:

- facts are external to us and can be discovered;
- the observing subject and observed object are separate and;
- observation of facts contributes to the development of theories in order to make generalizations.

The work setting can offer many ideas such as practices, problems and procedures which lend themselves to research, for example the evaluation of carers' needs, factors influencing presentation at services, attitudes of care providers, utilization by patients of a service or one of its branches, assessment of patient's motivation, adoption of a model to an area of care, assessment and measurement of change of behaviour or a prevalence study. Scrutiny of published research articles in the specialist journals and a search of the alcohol and drug research registers, which may be found in alcohol and drug reference libraries, can also assist to generate ideas. Discussion with and submission of the researcher's written views to the research supervisor will involve, and improve, the definition of the problem, suitability of the topic, testing of the theory to be explained, planning of the project and the methods of data collection and analysis. At this stage, beginning the drafting of a written proposal or protocol to contain these points will improve clarity, develop

Table 25.1 An approach to research

- Area of study
- Selection of topic
- Decide upon the methods to be used
- Formulate a plan
- Collect the data/information
- Analyse and interpret the findings
- Present the results

better conceptual and methodological skills as well as improving an ability to be critical and hence produce a better design of the research (Jairath and Fitch, 1994). A guide to the steps involved in research is described in Table 25.1

It would be expected that diploma and first degree projects would demonstrate some amount of analytical rigour, independent inquiry, exercise of judgement and a reasonable standard of presentation of the results (Howard and Sharp, 1989). Also, projects are usually governed by a size range which involve penalization if too short or too long.

All research should have a purpose and a project may be:

- a review or critique of an existing piece of research;
- a worked-out proposal of a larger project;
- a fully executed, small scale or pilot study.

The purpose can review, describe a situation, construct something new or seek to explain something. The fieldwork may consist of simple observation, secondary analysis of other documentation, experimentation, questionnaire and interview, policy evaluation, action research or ethnographic experiment. The aim may be to test a theory, to construct a new theory, to describe something or to specifically solve a problem. Data that consists mainly of words, sounds or images is termed qualitative and data consisting mainly of numbers are termed quantitative. The types of data generated by the fieldwork will determine the coding and tests to determine and define any association between the variables or attributes being studied.

A formal description of the written-up proposed study is known as the research proposal or protocol, and requires assembly in a standard manner. An outline of a proposal is contained in Table 25.2 and a fuller explanation and description can be found in Robertson (1994).

Again, the length and standard expected in the proposal will depend upon the level of the research, and one for a project such as a diploma will require a minimum of four to five double spaced A4 pages. It is generally expected that projects will be written and presented in a standardized format. Published guidelines covering the presentation of reports may be obtained from libraries, and these will also give methods of referencing and the presentation of bibliographies to bring the report to the level demanded.

Table 25.2 Description of research proposal

1 Project title

2 Introduction
  - incidence of problem
  - current level of knowledge
  - literature review
  - aim of the study, including key concepts
  - significance of the study

3 Method
  - study population
  - eligibility criteria, sampling size and rationale, control group
  - instrumentation for data collection
  - data analysis and approach
  - consent, ethical and administrative procedures
  - limitations of study
  - potential contribution to nursing knowledge

4 References

5 Appendices
  - consent form, data collection instruments, sample size calculations

A good and feasible research question is one that contains an amount of conceptual depth, showing that the researcher has understood the extent and nature of the task involved. A successful project is one that has been systematically planned and carried out in an ordered and logical sequence.

Future directions in research.

The last 20 years has seen considerable expansion and change in addiction services in line with the nature and extent of drug misuse and the policy changes prevailing upon subsequent responses and practices in the treatment of substance misuse. For addiction nurses, this presents numerous opportunities to undertake their own research. It is at the 'sharp end' of addiction treatment that most nurses are involved, that is at the point at which the service is delivered to the patient on a day-to-day basis. In this situation, the nurse wishing to undertake research is well placed to decide upon the purpose and nature of the study, being able to identify areas that would benefit from closer, systematic scrutiny.

The topic for research will of course be determined by numerous factors, such as the area in which the addiction nurse is working (community or in-patient services), any predetermined purpose of the research whether for an academic purpose such as a college project, or as part of a ward audit. Other elements such as time factors may also influence the length or content of any report.

There is a dearth of nursing research in addiction and therefore the potential field for addiction nursing research remains wide. Nurses working in custodial settings, non-statutory services, rehabilitation and detoxification units, within community or in-patient settings can all contribute to the general body of knowledge by researching and reporting on their own particular aspect. For example, looking at changes in local patterns of drug use and describing and attempting to account for changes, or reviewing the effectiveness of the treatment service (Wetherill *et al.*, 1987) should lie within the capabilities of most nurses. Our own practices, knowledge and beliefs could also provide suitable topics for nursing research, such as working with alcohol misusers in a general hospital setting (Leslie and Learmonth, 1994) and assessing the knowledge of HIV among health and social care professionals (Carroll, 1994).

Nurses are able to produce research. However, there should be an awareness of the potential for producing insular research along the lines of 'this is what we do on our ward'. Nursing research is sometimes criticized for being limited in scope, using too small a sample or lacking scientific approach. Possibly such work is interesting in its own right, but it can only contribute little to the core of nursing research.

What is not in question though is the value of the research nurse to the future of addiction nursing. As nursing strives to improve its professional standing, so too will it need to improve continually the academic and clinical rigour of its knowledge and skills base. Nursing research should be at the forefront of this drive, both in broadening the research base of nursing care and furthering the development of nursing science. This should permit the development of a greater number of research nurses being employed to carry out nursing research. This is an expense, but the acquisition of knowledge is costly – but much less so than ignorance.

CONCLUSION

While this chapter has introduced some of the issues presenting within addiction nursing and research, it does not claim to cover them all or offer all the answers. Research is increasingly being incorporated in the nursing remit and should be welcomed both as an essential part of personal professional development and enhancing the professional status of addiction nursing.

REFERENCES

Carroll, J. (1994) Professionals and drug users. *Nursing Standard*, **8**(43), 42–5.

Department of Health (1994) *Report of the Mental Health Nursing Review Team, Working in partnership*, HMSO, London.

Ghodse, A.H. (1977) Drug dependent individuals dealt with by London casualty departments. *British Journal of Psychiatry*, **131**, 273–80.

Howard, K. and Sharp, J.A. (1989) *The management of a student research project*, Gower, Aldershot.

Jairath, N. and Fitch, M. (1994) The Generic Research Protocol: an innovative technique to facilitate research skills development and protocol preparation. *The Journal of Continuing Education in Nursing*, **25**(3), 111–14.

Leslie, H. and Learmonth, L. (1994) Alcohol counselling in a general hospital. *Nursing Standard*, **8**(27), 25–9.

MacGregor, S., Ettore, B., Coomber, R., Crosier, A. and Lodge, L. (1991) *Drug services in England and the impact of the central funding initiative*, Institute for the Study of Drug Dependence, London.

Robertson, J. (ed) (1994) *Handbook of clinical nursing research*, Churchill Livingstone, Edinburgh.

Smith, L. (1992) Ethical issues in interviewing. *Journal of Advanced Nursing*, **17**(1), 98–103.

Tober, G. (1994) Drug taking in a northern UK city. *Accident & Emergency Nursing*, **2**(2), 70–8.

Wetherill, J., Kelly, T. and Hore, B. (1987) The role of the community psychiatric nurse in improving treatment compliance in alcoholics. *Journal of Advanced Nursing*, **12**(6), 707–11.

Appendix A

EDUCATION AND TRAINING RESOURCES

Anglia Polytechnic University
Faculty of Health & Social Work
Broomfield Hospital
Chelmsford
Essex GMI 5LG
England
Tel: 01245 440334 Fax: 01245 443034

Diploma of Credit in Substance Misuse (ENB)

Aquarius Education Training and Consultancy
6th Floor
The White House
111 New Street
Birmingham B2 4EU
England
Tel: 0121 632 4727 Fax: 0121 633 0539

HIT (formerly the Mersey Drug Training and Information Centre)
Cavern Walks
8 Mathew Street
Liverpool L2 6RE
England
Tel: 0151 227 4012 Fax: 0151 227 4023

Leeds Addiction Unit
19 Springfield Mount
Leeds LS2 9NG
England
Tel: 0113 2926930 Fax: 0113 292 6950

Diploma in Substance Misuse (ENB)

Liverpool John Moores University
Social and Human Sciences Department
Trueman Building
15–21 Webster Street
Liverpool L3 2ET
England
Tel: 0151 231 4029 Fax: 0151 258 1224

Maudsley/Regional Drug Training Unit Diploma in Drug Dependence
National Addiction Centre   (ENB)
4 Windsor Walk
Camberwell
London SE5 8AF
England
Tel: 0171 703 0269 Fax: 0171 703 0269

Redwood College of Health Studies/   Recognition and Management of
South Bank University   Substance Misuse (ENB)
Education Centre
Harold Wood Hospital
Gubbins Lane
Harold Wood
Romford RM3 0BE.
England
Tel: 0171 815 5959 Fax: 0171 815 5906

Ruskin College   Certificate in Multidisciplinary
Dunstan Hall   Studies of Drug Use
Old Headington
Oxford OX3 9BZ
England
Tel: 01865 63437 Fax: 01793 825583

South West Drugs Training Service
National Association Care and Resettlement of Offenders (NACRO)
29 A Southgate
Bath BA1 1TP
England
Tel: 01225 336766 Fax: 01225 466495.

St George's Hospital Medical School
Department of Addictive Behaviour
Centre for Addiction Studies
(University of London)
Hunter Wing
Cranmer Terrace
Tooting
London SW16 0RE
England
Tel: 0181 725 2637 Fax: 0181 725 2914

Certificate in Substance Misuse (ENB)
Diploma in Addictive Behaviour
(ENB)
MSc in Addictive Behaviour

The Centre for Research and Health Behaviour
200 Seagrave Road
London SW6 1RQ
England
Tel: 0181 846 6565 Fax: 0181 846 6555

Certificate in Drug and Alcohol
Studies
Diploma in Drug and Alcohol Studies
(ENB)

University of Kent
School of Continuing Education
Keynes College
Canterbury
Kent CT2 7NP
England
Tel 0227 764000 Fax: 01227 458745

Diploma in Alcohol Counselling and
Consultation

University of Nottingham
School of Nursing and Midwifery
B Floor
Queen's Medical Centre
Nottingham NG7 2UH
England
Tel: 0115 924 9924 Fax: 0115 942 3876

Drug & Alcohol Dependency (ENB)

University of Paisley
Centre for Alcohol and Drug Studies
Westerfield House
25 High Calside
Paisley PA2 6BY
Scotland
Tel: 0141 848 3141 Fax: 0141 848 3000

Postgraduate Diploma in Alcohol
studies

University of Stirling
Drugs Training Project
Department of Sociology
Stirling FK9 4LE
Scotland
Tel: 0176 467732 Fax: 01786 467979

West Midlands Regional Drugs Training Unit
6 Unity Place
Albert Street
Oldbury
West Midlands B69 4DD
England
Tel: 0121 544 3939 Fax: 0121 544 2094

Appendix B

ORGANIZATIONS: INFORMATION AND RESOURCES

Action on Smoking and Health (ASH)
109 Gloucester Place
London W1H 4EJ
England
Tel: 0171 935 3519 Fax: 0171 935 3463

Addiction Research Foundation (ARF)
32 Russell Street
Ontario M5S 2S1
Canada
Tel: 416 595 6000

Alcohol Action Wales/Gweithredu Alcohol Cymru
4 Dock Chambers
Bute Street
Cardiff CF1 6AG
Wales
Tel/Ffon: 01222 4888000 Fax/Ffacs: 01222 488000

Alcohol Concern
Waterbridge House
32–36 Loman Street
London SE1 0EE
England
Tel: 0171 928 7377 Fax: 0171 928 4644

Alcohol Education and Research Council
Room 143
Horseferry House
Dean Ryle Street
London SW1P 2AH
England
Tel: 0171 217 8393

Association of Nurses in Substance Abuse (ANSA)
Professional Briefings
120 Wilton Road
London SW1V 1JZ
England
Tel: 0171 233 8322 Fax: 0171 233 7779

Centre for Addiction Studies
Department of Addictive Behaviour
St George's Hospital Medical School, (University of London)
Hunter Wing, Cranmer Terrace
Tooting, London SW16 0RE
England
Tel: 0181 725 2637 Fax: 0181 725 2914

Drug and Alcohol Nurse Association (DANA)
660 Lonely College Drive
Upper Black Eddy
PA 18972–9313
USA

European Association for the Treatment of Addiction (EATA) (UK)
6th Floor, 25–27 Oxford Street
London W1R 1RF
England
Tel: 0171 439 3229 Fax: 0171 494 1764

Health Education Authority
Hamilton House
Mabledon Place
London WC1A 9TY
England
Tel: 0171 383 3833

Health Education Board for Scotland
Wooburn House
Canaan Lane
Edinburgh
Scotland
Tel: 0131 447 6180 Fax: 0131 452 8140

Health Promotion Agency for Northern Ireland
18 Ormeau Avenue
Belfast BT2 8HS
Northern Ireland
Tel: 01232 311611 Fax: 01232 311711

Health Promoton Wales/Hybu Iechyd Cymru
Ffynnon-las
Ty Glas Avenue
Llanishen
Cardiff
Wales
Tel/ Ffon: 01222 752222
Fax/Ffacs: 01222 756000

Institute for the Study of Drug Dependence
Waterbridge House
32–36 Loman Street
London SE1 0EE
England
Tel: 0171 928 1211 Fax: 0171 928 7071

International Council on Alcohol and Addictions (ICAA)
Case Postale 189
1001 Lausanne
Switzerland
Tel: 021 320 98 65

National Addiction Centre
4 Windsor Walk
Camberwell
London SE5 8AF
England
Tel: 0171 703 5411 Fax: 0171 919 2171

National Drug and Alcohol Research Centre
University of New South Wales
PO Box 1
Kensington NSW2033
Australia
Tel: 02 398 9333

National Institute of Alcohol Abuse (NIAA)
5600 Fishers Lane
Rockville MD 20857
USA
Tel: (301) 443 3885

National Institute of Drug Abuse (NIDA)
5600 Fishers Lane
Rockville MD 20857
USA
Tel: (301) 443 6480

National Nurses Society on Addiction (NNSA)
5700 Old Orchard Road
Skokie IL 60077
USA
Tel: (708) 966 5010.

Northern Ireland Council on Alcohol
40 Elmwood Avenue
Belfast BT9 6A2
Northern Ireland
Tel: 01232 664434 Fax: 01232 664090

Office for Substance Abuse Prevention
National Clearing-House for Alcohol and Drug Information (NCADI)
PO Box 2345
Rockville
Maryland 20852 USA
Tel: 301 468 2600

RCN Substance Misuse Forum
Royal College Of Nursing
20 Cavendish Square
London W1M 0AB
England
Tel: 0171 409 3333 Fax: 0171 409 1379

Scottish Council on Alcohol (SCA)
2nd Floor
166 Buchanan Street
Glasgow G1 2NH
Scotland
Tel: 0141 333 9677 Fax: 0141 333 1606

Scottish Drug Forum
5 Oswald Street
Glasgow G1 4QR
Scotland
Tel: 0141 221 1175 Fax: 0141 248 6414

Society for the Study of Addiction to Alcohol and Other Drugs
Department of Forensic Psychiatry
Institute of Psychiatry
De Crespigny Park
London SE5 8AF
England
Tel: 0171 703 5411 Fax: 0171 277 0283

Standing Conference on Drug Abuse (SCODA)
Waterbridge House
32–36 Loman Street
London SE1 0EE
England
Tel: 0171 928 9500 Fax: 0171 928 3343

The Advisory Council on Alcohol and Drug Education (TACADE)
1 Humle Place
The Crescent
Salford
Manchester
England
Tel: 0161 745 8925 Fax: 0161 745 8923

World Health Organization (WHO)
CH-1211
Geneva 27
Switzerland
Tel: 22 791 2111 Fax: 22 791 0746

Index

Page numbers in *italic* refer to tables